Complementary Therapies in the
Care of Older People

Dedication

To my husband Cliff with love and thanks for everything.

Complementary Therapies in the Care of Older People

HELEN BRETT MSc, RN, DipN(Lon)

Senior Lecturer, Faculty of Health,
Canterbury Christ Church University College, Canterbury

W

WHURR PUBLISHERS
LONDON AND PHILADELPHIA

© 2002 Whurr Publishers
First published 2002 by
Whurr Publishers Ltd
19b Compton Terrace, London N1 2UN, England and
325 Chestnut Street, Philadelphia PA 19106, USA

Reprinted 2003

British Library Cataloguing in Publication Data
A catalogue record for this book is available from the British
Library.

ISBN: 1 86156 304 3

Contents

The author

Helen Brett MSc, RN, DipN(Lon), Cert Ed, is a Senior Lecturer at Canterbury Christ Church University College. She has a certificate in Anatomy, Physiology and Massage (ITEC), a Certificate in Reflex Zone Therapy (IEB for IFR), and a diploma in Holistic Aromatherapy (ISPA), and is a Practising Member of the International Society of Professional Aromatherapists and an Associate Member of the British Acupuncture Register.

Foreword

Individuals' reactions to the subject of complementary therapies differ greatly. For some, such therapy is an essential part of their treatment or vital to the maintenance of their wellbeing, while the opinion of others ranges from mild interest to hearty scepticism. Clearly, knowledge, experience and hearsay may influence people's views. Complementary therapy encompasses a broad portfolio of activities and it is important to clarify the various components, to give them meaning and to explain their scope in practice. This timely book provides the key to an understanding of the reality of complementary therapies and dispels many myths. It is primarily concerned with older people but some aspects of the therapies are applicable to other groups.

Any therapy requires permission from the receiver or their agent; to proceed otherwise is a violation of the individual's human rights as well as likely to reduce the value of the intervention. This is of crucial importance in complementary therapy techniques that use touch as a medium. Elderly people may be particularly concerned about touch. While a conventional handshake from a comparative stranger can be acceptable, many people find any other contact is a highly objectional intrusion.

Our health services have experienced major changes, which have affected the way in which patient care is delivered. In some instances these factors have led to a reduction in the direct contact element of professional care, particularly in nursing. Many nurses seek to address this for the benefit of patients and for their own job enrichment. Complementary therapies provide an opportunity for this.

For such therapy to be successful a practical approach is needed and this requires two interlinked aspects – 'Manner' and 'Method'.

Manner applies to all physical and verbal human communication; its presence promotes a successful outcome to intervention and the converse is true. Manner includes: the therapist's general presentation and approach to the patient and others; the clarity and level of the explanation given; a statement of objectives of the treatment; the securing of agreement from the patient; the provision of a safe environment.

Method includes information about the range of therapies available, details of their applicability, the balance between them, their efficacy and the evidence on which their use is based.

This book covers many aspects of 'Manner' and 'Method' and presents them in a comprehensive way. It takes a holistic approach, balancing complementary therapies with conventional treatments; it deals with sensitive subjects ably and clearly. The inclusion of actual cases is a helpful way of applying the subject matter. The author is a very experienced professional person who shares her knowledge, skill and caring attitude with the reader. Practising nurses and other professionals will find this text a mine of information. It will also be valuable to elderly persons and their carers since it gives possible scenarios that may affect them and identifies potential sources of help.

When formal or informal carers are planning care, the patient's individual needs must be considered. In determining the care to be given, a range of options should be explored. *Complementary Therapies in the Care of Older People* considerably increases that range. This knowledge helps us to be creative in our care and permits us to develop innovative practice.

Peta Allan
October 2001

Preface

I have written this book to provide you with an insight into using complementary therapies safely with older people. Although I have written it primarily for nurses, I hope it may also be of interest to other carers, patients or older people themselves. I have tried to provide the information in a lively way and have drawn heavily on my experiences as both a complementary practitioner and a nurse lecturer, still very actively concerned with the care of older people (I have been the module leader for ENB 941 for the past 10 years). The therapies I have chosen to include in this book are those in which I am qualified and experienced, and that also happen to be those that are most commonly used by nurses.

As a result of the controversies and assorted issues surrounding the use of complementary therapies, the foremost aim of this book must be to introduce you to safe and realistic practice. Therefore, alongside the theoretical component, I have given examples of how such therapies can be integrated into current nursing care. I also show clearly when it is inadvisable to pursue this option! As you read I hope you will be critical and challenge the content, because is not my intention to teach you all you need to know about these therapies, but to help raise your awareness of the joys and pitfalls of using such therapies within orthodox settings. Because of this, at the end of some of the chapters I have posed questions, although in others I have used an interactive and somewhat more provocative language, to stimulate you into thinking about just how you might offer patients and carers the choice of enjoying complementary therapies, either partly or in their entirety.

I have greatly enjoyed the opportunity given to me by Whurr Publishers of putting this book together, and it has encouraged me to journey even further along this road of discovery, especially as His Royal Highness The Prince of Wales, an advocate of integrated medicine, asserts:

> It is no longer a question of hacking a path through unexplored jungle. The way is landmarked, the goals and prizes are visible. All that is needed is courage -- and a little imagination.
>
> Editorial (2000)

I hope you, as nurses, may also benefit from some of the thoughts within this book, and I wish you good luck with any future endeavours. You may need it!

Helen Brett
October 2001

Reference

Editorial (2000) The way forward. His Royal Highness The Prince of Wales. Complementary Therapies in Nursing and Midwifery 6: 1–3.

Acknowledgements

I should like, first, to thank all those patients, clients and their families who have so generously allowed me to use their experiences to illustrate this book and also the nurses, managers, doctors, students and teaching colleagues who have helped me along the way.

Second, I would like to thank my husband and parents for their unending encouragement.

Special thanks must go to the following:

- my daughter Katharine Stowers for her constant support, computing advice and photography;
- my son Philip Stowers for his advice and making time to draw the illustrations;
- Sharon Barker, a former post-registration student, for her willingness to give openly of her continence expertise and share some of my journey (see Chapter 10);
- Peta Allan for kindly consenting to write the foreword;
- The Editorial Board of the International Society of Professional Aromatherapists (ISPA) for kindly giving permission to reproduce the case study, Alzheimer's disease (first published in *Aromatherapy World* (1997) Distillation, pp 31–33) (see Chapter 12);
- and finally, the team at Whurr Publishers who have given continual support and shown belief in me.

PART I

Considerations for safe practice

This part aims not only to set the scene and introduce you to the complexities and debate surrounding the introduction of complementary therapies into orthodox settings for elderly people, but also to give you the opportunity to consider touch and its appropriate use. An appreciation of both is essential, because these two facets form the basis of much of what is to follow.

CHAPTER 1

Integrating complementary therapies into the nursing care of older people

The need to address the many health problems faced by large numbers of older people everywhere increases daily. Ageing is an intricate and complex process that has been surrounded by myths and conjecture. Elderly people are hospitalised rarely and, when they are, it is usually because of some precipitating illness rather than just because they are old. Even non-specific symptoms tend to have some pathological cause. It has been said that old age is a gift of modern technology and that people are actually staying older rather than younger longer. Although it is imperative to differentiate between normal and pathological ageing, this increased lifespan has implications for care.

There have been various estimates made about the increases of numbers of older people. The World Health Organization (World Health Report 1997) stated that by 2002 this population would increase by 10% in developing countries and 40% in industrialised countries. The Royal Commission on Long Term Care (1999) reported that, by 2050, it is likely that there will be three times more people aged over 85 years than there are now. Henwood (1992) suggests that more than 50% of our population will be over 75 by 2041. However, the notion of the 'demographic time bomb' waiting to go off has been somewhat dispelled, because:

> . . . demographic pressures [have been] overstated. Over the next decade the NHS
> expects to provide services for an extra 100,000 aged 85 and over; but that is just one
> third of the increase it has coped with over the last decade.
>
> Department of Health (1997)

There are therefore still issues surrounding the care of this population that need to be addressed.

What do you think some of these issues might be?

Currently, although older people are major users of the health services in the UK, there is evidence to suggest that they are not well served by them (Health Advisory Service [HAS] 1997, 1998). Increasingly concerns have been raised, not only about the quality and level of health and social care provision being funded, but also about the lack of specialist gerontological nurses available to care for this 'greying population' (News 1996). It has been mooted that, if the health difficulties experienced by older people do not receive due attention, individuals and society may be culpable of both degrading elderly people and betraying their own ideals.

Do you think that complementary therapies have a role to play in this and why?

Holistic nursing recognises that patients have their own beliefs about health and hospitals and their own way of handling situations, and thus acknowledges the need to promote patient autonomy and the right to make an informed choice (Goodman 1995). Rankin-Box (1991) claims that the use of alternative therapies in nursing implies a shift in the locus of control from the carer to the recipient, thus providing for more patient autonomy.

Sidell (1995) thought that, broadly speaking, alternative therapies could offer older people the following:

- symptomatic relief from painful conditions
- care rather than cure
- could also help them cope with the emotional burden of loss.

As a result of this Sidell believed that there was some potential in using them, because they seemed more sensitive and congruent to the needs of older people. But she had two concerns about the provision of complementary therapies. First, she felt that they might be financially untenable for most older people because they are normally provided within the private sector, and second, that there are still some practitioners providing unregulated therapies for purely financial gain. Does this last statement just reflect the scepticism that sometimes surrounds these practitioners?

Fulder (1988) identified five basic characteristics of alternative therapies:

1. They explore and investigate any deficits and aim to restore the consequent imbalances.

2. They consider all aspects of the patient's world so that barriers that prevent treating the person as a whole are broken down.
3. Treatment is based on a much wider concept of health.
4. They are well suited to help chronic and degenerative, mental and physical disease processes and to aid self-healing.
5. They are mostly safe and non-toxic.

What are complementary therapies?

Can you formulate an adequate and acceptable definition?

Complementary therapies are often identified in terms of what they are not, rather than what they actually are. With more than 300 different techniques and modalities available, it is very easy to lose sight of the massive scope of these therapies and the potential problems for those seeking another type of care. Davis (1997) says that alternative and complementary therapies are based on different cultural beliefs and attitudes to orthodox medicine, especially when treating chronic illness and for preventive and health-promoting strategies, and have caused a massive change to occur in the health care of the industrialised West.

Although some therapies appear to have stood the test of time and are regulated, others are not and often have no proven efficacy or recognition. Although the general public tends to view them positively, some orthodox practitioners, who may feel threatened by the existence of other treatment modalities, may not because they believe that complementary therapies are unscientific and potentially harmful. For those who are attempting to provide complementary therapies, there is therefore a huge responsibility on them to provide adequate information and above all safe and effective practice.

Complementary therapies have been narrowly defined as:

> . . . those [therapies] which can work alongside and in conjunction with orthodox medical treatment.
>
> British Medical Association (1993)

Attempts have been made to classify these broad-ranging therapies. Bell and Sikora (1996), while recognizing that there was some inevitable overlap between categories, divided them into three main headings.

1. Psychological: these included not only the easily recognised therapies, such as counselling, psychotherapy, healing and visualisation, but also the more unusual ones such as radionics, psychic surgery and rebirthing.

2. Physical: this group contained possibly the most well-known therapies and listed massage, aromatherapy, reflexology, acupuncture and chiropractic.
3. Pharmacological: these seemed to include the most obscure therapies such as shark's cartilage and immunostimulation, although they did also record homoeopathy and dietary intervention.

Others such as Pietroni (1992), however, classified them according to how they may be used and listed them under four broad headings:

1. Complete systems, which included acupuncture and osteopathy.
2. Diagnostic methods such as iridology and hair analysis.
3. Therapeutic modalities, which included aromatherapy, massage and reflexology.
4. Self-care approaches such as meditation, yoga and relaxation.

The phrase 'complementary therapy' is therefore just an umbrella term that covers the broad range of treatments available. Although the term 'alternative' is commonly used, other terms such as natural, unorthodox and unconventional are also used and, although they are all closely related, they are not necessarily synonymous.

Complementary versus alternative therapies

The two major terms used, 'complementary' and 'alternative', are often perceived in very different ways. Complementary is seen as something that can be used alongside another therapy in order to enhance a treatment, but the word 'alternative' is perceived as purely an alternative to orthodox treatment. Yet, Davis (1997) notes how the terms are often used interchangeably. The word 'alternative' does appear to imply something negative and less worthy, and perhaps it is this term that has impeded the growth of other therapies, alongside orthodox medicine.

In an article entitled 'Alternative roads to hell?', Gennis (1992), an Evangelical Christian, wrote rather emotively, about their use, but she seems to have confused such therapies with the 'New Age' movement. She evidently believes strongly that therapies that purport to heal go against Christian thinking, especially when their underlying philosophies are imbued with pagan traditions. She is also concerned that Christian patients may be being duped, because when they are offered some of these alternative treatments they may not realise that the inherent values of these therapies are very different from those they hold dear. Uncomfortable as it may be, there may be an element of truth in this.

Sutcliffe (2001) also recognizes that some churches regard complementary therapies with suspicion but, as a practising Christian and aromatherapist herself, she believes that they may have a poor understanding of some of the therapies and, as a consequence of this, labelled them, like Gennis (1992) as 'weird, satanic, or occult'. She feels that complementary therapies do have a place, alongside orthodox medicine, in the care of patients but she says that they must not be used to:

... shift focus from prayer and faith [or as a] substitute for trust in the Lord.

She clarifies her Christian position further, by noting that:

God gave us all good things for our use [and] – although He gave our bodies the ability to heal themselves, sometimes healing needs physical help – from both conventional medical treatments and more natural complementary therapies. The final word is proceed with caution.

Prince Charles in a guest editorial (Editorial 2000) stated that over the years the National Health Service (NHS) had mostly thought of complementary medicine as 'fringe' or even 'quack' medicine and had found it an 'uncomfortable bedfellow'. He added that he had been encouraged that the British Medical Association (BMA) were now less sceptical of his belief in such therapies than when he spoke to them 16 years earlier. He felt that this had been markedly influenced by the general public's growing appreciation of them.

Peace and Simmons (1996) also noticed a change of heart in the language of the two BMA reports. The first (BMA 1986) was critical of alternative therapies and stressed that any benefits they might bring were purely the result of the placebo effect. Their second report (BMA 1993) was couched in much softer terms, possibly because doctors, by then, had also recognised that more and more patients were seeking them out. It therefore justly called for: more research into the efficacy of complementary medicine; the development of postgraduate courses to inform doctors about such therapies; and single regulation of each therapy before they could become a part of mainstream health care.

This shift in vocabulary may aid recognition of such philosophies, especially as Peace and Simmons (1996) argue that complementary merely means that which when added complements the whole. Yet some therapists may argue that there is a need for an alternative to orthodox medicine, such as the traditional Chinese medicine (TCM) system of care, and that the use of the word complementary is purely used to make it easier for other health professionals to accept such therapies. Wright (1995) notes how at one time the word alternative predominated, but that the terminology has now been moderated so that nurses may be able to get the necessary support to use them within their nursing practice. He, like Kendrick (1999), thinks this is a mere concession so that it will be more acceptable to other healthcare professionals!

Consider why it might be preferable for nurses to use the term 'complementary' when looking at integrating therapies into practice.

More recently the term CAM (complementary and alternative medicine) has been adopted within the literature and has been defined as:

> . . . diagnosis, treatment and/or prevention which complements mainstream medicine by contributing to a common whole, by satisfying a demand not met by orthodoxy or by the conceptual frameworks of medicine.
>
> Ernst and Cassileth (1998)

Why is this a better title?

Increase in popularity of complementary therapies

Identify some of the factors that have led to an increase in the popularity and usage of complementary therapies over the last two decades.

Over the last 25 years complementary therapies have rapidly grown in popularity (Eisenberg et al. 1998). A survey conducted by the National Association of Health Authorities and Trusts (1993) showed that £1m of public money was spent on purchasing complementary treatments in 1993; this is generally recognised as a gross underestimate given that it included less than half of the health districts and did not take into account the less formal, non-contractual arrangements for complementary therapies. The European COST Report (European Commission 1998) identified other factors that might account for this rise in interest. Unfortunately, some of the reasons given were because of mistrust, dissatisfaction and disillusionment with not only orthodox medicine, but its practitioners as well. It did, however, also highlight that complementary therapies allowed a more respectful and open approach to care.

BBC Radio 5 Live Survey (Ernst and White 2000)

There is very little information about the use of complementary therapies by the general public in the UK, although it has been estimated that four to five million people a year in the UK consult a complementary practitioner. Stone (1999) felt that this was quite remarkable as most people fund these treatments themselves. A large study of Eisenberg et al. (1998), which was conducted between 1990 and 1997, found that the use of CAM within the USA had increased from 33% to 42%. As most of the statistics available about the use of complementary therapies relate mostly to American and Australian populations, in the summer of 1999 Radio 5 Live commissioned ICM research to:

> . . . determine the use of CAM in the UK general population.
>
> Ernst and White (2000)

The study details

Adults, over the age of 18 years, were interviewed by telephone and were asked five questions. No record was kept of those who declined to answer. A total of 1204 interviews were conducted over 2 days.

The results showed the following:

- Twenty per cent (a fifth) noted that they had used CAM positively over the last year.
- Six per cent said that someone they knew had used CAM.
- Women aged between 35 and 64 years used them the most.
- They were mostly used in Wales (32%) and south-east England (23%).
- Most of the sample used aromatherapy, massage reflexology, herbalism, acupuncture, acupressure, homoeopathy, but also used flower remedies, osteopathy, healing, etc.
- Seventy-eight per cent felt that CAM use was increasing and 8 felt no change. The respondents felt that this increase was as a result of users liking CAM because they perceived them to be a useful aid to relaxation and also because they were effective.
- The respondents estimated that they spent between £5 and £13 per month on them (the researchers urged caution about these figures as they suggested that people tend not to remember accurately how much they spend).

Although it is not easy to compare either across countries or between surveys because the terminology for such therapies is often expressed quite differently, this survey is highly suggestive of an increased use within the UK. For future surveys, it may be preferable to discover more specifically what therapy is being used for which conditions and discover just how efficacious, safe and cost-effective they are.

The reasons for this prolific increase in use are felt to arise from the common philosophies and themes that differentiate CAM from conventional medicine. The relationship between the mind, body and spirit, the holistic approach and the individual's interaction with the environment set CAM apart from the traditional Cartesian science-based approach, and this appears to be particularly appealing to those people who suffer from chronic illnesses and stress-related disorders. This may be because its focus is on the person, promoting well-being and restoring energy and balance, and not purely about curing.

Given this steady rise in the popularity of complementary therapies, it is not surprising that in some areas there are growing tensions with regard to its use, lack of regulation, indeterminate standards and comparatively little research into its effectiveness.

Disillusionment and disenchantment with allopathic medicine and the growth of other therapies probably arose because people wanted help from other sources instead of having to rely totally on medical and surgical initiatives (more will be said in Chapter 15 about this).

There is tremendous debate within the literature as to whether or not complementary therapies are holistic, but Sidell (1995) feels that nurses may be adopting them because they believe that holism is their underlying philosophy. Long et al. (2000) suspect that there is some evidence to support this notion, although it is a concept that is very difficult to measure. Although not suggesting in any way that allopathic medicine is a non-holistic practice, by developing a sensitive measure it may be possible to determine the extent to which such therapies are holistic and also to determine that what is being measured is part of the process of treatment, rather than just an outcome of care.

Buckle (1993), however, firmly believes that complementary therapies are no more holistic than orthodox therapies unless nurses take on their fundamental philosophies as well. She adds that, as holism only means being a whole, in order that we do care for people 'wholly' all aspects such as the spiritual and the physical must be encompassed within our care. She therefore asserts that:

> . . . if it is true that patients need to reach out in their hour of crisis in an attempt to become finally 'whole' [then] we need holism rather than complementary therapies . . .

because without looking after the total needs of the patient we are only practising another therapy.

Even so, Siddell (1995) says that medicine is still deeply suspicious of such therapies, although complementary practitioners counteract this argument by pointing out that biomedicine is imposing its own method of scientific proof on alternative therapy, which is wholly inappropriate because the goals of the two forms of treatment are different. Alongside the growth in popularity is the growing need for a sustained research base. Much of the criticism levelled at the complementary field by conventionalist medicine is associated with increasing anxiety regarding treatment efficacy and safety.

So, how can these therapies be integrated into nursing practice?
What are the potential benefits they might bring to your patients?
Are there any pitfalls?

There is increasing evidence that the public is now more interested in and indeed seeking out complementary, as opposed to orthodox, approaches to care (Foundation for Integrated Medicine 1997). Although many nurses appear eager to introduce some of these methods into their patients' care (Stevenson 1994), they often encounter considerable problems when they try to do this (Rankin-Box 1997). Although the therapies have grown in importance over the last two decades, to date there appear to be only two studies that have sought to canvas nurses' views on what they feel about and how they use different therapies (Rankin-Box 1997, Trevelyan 1998). It would seem that, although nurses are using a variety of mostly tactile therapies, these are mostly used within private practice and not as part of everyday care within the NHS (Rankin-Box 1997). It is primarily lone nurses, working unaided, who are battling to integrate them into their everyday nursing care (Brett 1999).

Complementary therapies have the potential to add another dimension to the care of older patients and, although there is a vast array from which nurses may choose, it seems that the most common ones used are the touch therapies, such as massage and aromatherapy. I would like to add just a word of caution before you enthusiastically embrace these concepts. The patients for whom you care are a very vulnerable, captive population and, in order that they may experience the safest of care, it is essential for you to be aware of the following. Although these therapies are increasingly sought after and seen to be desirable to use, there have been some concerns expressed about both the validity of the therapies and the therapist's ability to offer them effectively. Therefore before introducing any non-orthodox therapies to your client group you must: abide by your Code of Professional Conduct (UKCC 1992a); obtain relevant medical and managerial permission; and also obtain fully informed consent from your patients and then practise competently.

To integrate alternative therapies into nursing practice, it is vital to know not only that they are benefiting the patient, but also by how much and which conditions respond more positively to one therapy than another, thus validating further therapies and enabling funds and resources to be more effectively allocated (Rankin-Box 1991). Good (1995) suggests that documentation of findings, such as with the use of pain charts to show potential benefits of relaxation and visualisation therapies, could be one example of a way in which we could evaluate effectiveness and enhance the credibility of our practice. Equally, however, acceptance and involvement are needed from all staff to ensure continuity and success of this different practice. This may not be easy to achieve, however.

Resistance, especially from medical staff, is often attributed to the belief that they are trapped inside a model that rigidly separates physical from emotional events, and are therefore distrustful of any practice that claims to treat both (Kiddel 1986). Choosing an alternative healthcare practice, even while receiving treatment in a biomedical setting, can be seen by doctors as non-compliance on the part of the patient or as a strategy to gain control of the patient themselves (Montbriand 1991).

Consider specific ways in which you could safely integrate therapies into your practice area

The process for safe integration of therapies

Before introducing these complementary therapies into any clinical area, there must be a clear policy supported by a rationale for using the chosen therapy/therapies. This policy should promote and classify principles of practice and be directed at safeguarding the patient and the public (McVey 1996). All policy developments should reinforce the United Kingdom Central Council (UKCC) guidelines associated with professional accountability and assist the nurse towards identifying competent practice to avoid compromising her or his professional practice (UKCC 1992a). If the therapy is to be provided by a complementary therapist, who is not a nurse or part of the ward team, other policies will apply.

Even though consultation with medical practitioners and nursing and trust management is paramount when establishing a policy, a survey carried out by the NHS Confederation in 1997 found that trusts that attempted to develop policies identified a number of barriers to this. The two most difficult to overcome were: objections to the use of other therapies by doctors and lack of senior nurse management support. This lack of support made it much more difficult for these policy proposals to be adopted than those involving more conventional services (Trevelyan 1998a).

Wafer (1994) stressed that any new innovation should be introduced only if it is realistic to practise, helpful and safe for the patient, and complements current orthodox care. Wafer (1994) noted how, in his hospital, there was a growing awareness of complementary therapies and alongside this the need to develop skills in therapies such as massage and aromatherapy. He also felt that there was an urgent need to develop written guidelines about their specific use within orthodox settings. These guidelines for aromatherapy were developed by a small working party and they recommended not only safe administration of therapies but also sufficient educational input to inform this.

It is, however, difficult to establish these, as in the *Guidelines for the Administration of Medicines* (UKCC 2000, page 9) there is only one brief paragraph, which states:

Complementary and alternative therapies are increasingly used in the treatment of patients. Registered nurses, midwives and health visitors who practise the use of such therapies must have successfully undertaken training and be competent in this area (please refer to the scope of professional practice). You must have considered the appropriateness of the therapy to both the condition of the patient and any coexisting treatments. It is essential that the patient is aware of the therapy and gives informed consent.

Although this statement begs many questions about competence, etc. and also about how judgements in the light of current available knowledge can be made, it does seem to be the ideal base from which to develop a protocol. Although, not speaking specifically about complementary therapies, Naish's (1997) guidance relating to the development of new roles is invaluable. He notes that the UKCC supports the notion of protocols when nurses are undertaking work previously done by doctors and lists S Dowling's (unpublished at that time) recommendations for reducing nurse risk and vulnerability when adopting new roles, all of which could so easily apply to the nurse taking on another therapist's role instead. They include ensuring that the new role is clearly defined, that accountability arrangements and level of competence are agreed, and that all involved, including the patients, understand them. He added that to ensure their success there also needs to be effective management to provide support and focus, especially early on when the changes and adaptation necessary to expand these new role are at their greatest.

Clause 9.4 of *The Scope of Professional Practice* (UKCC 1992b, page 6), however, clearly states that each registered nurse, midwife or health visitor:

> . . . must ensure that any enlargement or adjustment of the scope of personal professional practice must be achieved without compromising or fragmenting existing aspects of professional practice and care and that the requirements of the Council's Code of Professional Conduct [1992a] are satisfied throughout the whole area of practice.

Not all nurses have found this document (UKCC 1992b) useful and a recent article, 'Fitness for practice' (Anon 2001b), notes that, although some nurses are welcoming more flexibility in their role, others are not keen to lose the security afforded to them by the extended role certificates of the past. Although they recognised that, in order to practise new skills, they would be expected to undertake some training, they felt that the guidance given was not specific enough to protect future endeavours. To provide nurses with adequate protection, it is clear that firm proposals and protocols do need to be developed before embarking on any therapy introduction.

Proposals and protocols

Any proposal (Anon 1999) must be based on a systematic assessment of need and evidence-based practice. The Foundation for Integrated Medicine (FIM 1997) suggest that any proposal should therefore focus on:

- Areas of need that could be better served by complementary therapies than current nursing practice.
- Specific conditions, which are treated efficaciously by complementary therapies.

They could possibly be integrated in the following three ways:

1. Being introduced as a service in its own right, e.g. a clinic offering a specialist service such as aromatherapy. Although it may be hard to justify funding such as a broad-based service, consideration is more likely to be given to initiatives (such as 2 and 3 below) arising out of individual patient need, especially if they can be seen as potential therapeutic nursing interventions that have incorporated new evidence into their development.

2. Being focused on a particular health need, e.g. introducing relaxation within a support group for patients suffering interstitial cystitis (Brett and Barker 1998).
3. Developing professional nursing practice in a specific clinical area, i.e. using aromatherapy hand massage (Brett 1999).

The proposal

The proposal must clearly differentiate between what a nurse is able to provide and what a complementary therapist may provide. You also need to be able to describe exactly what will be offered (Brett 1999). This initial document needs to be well presented, objective and realistic, especially in relation to resourcing issues. In addition to this, it needs to identify clearly the objectives, scope of service and clinical rationale for the changes planned. Your action plan must include issues of quality, safety, consent, competence to practice, and accountability and risk management. It should also highlight constraints and implications for colleagues and collaborative working. If there is not already a protocol in existence, one needs to be formulated.

Do not be deterred by this but just remember:

> . . . nurses trying to introduce change within the confines of an NHS setting need to realize that unless they are fully committed to the idea, the lengthy consultation and implementation period could act as a deterrent.
>
> Brett (1999)

Trevelyan (1998a) believes that, because senior managers are not very interested in providing complementary services, it is normally harder for nurses who wish to do so to get their proposals accepted. You have been warned!

As I often provide introductory sessions on the safe use of complementary therapies to various people, I have found the following aide-mémoire invaluable (Table 1.1). It is short and succinct and encompasses all aspects that a nurse must consider before using them alongside orthodox practice.

Safe practice

It will be useful to look at this safe practice aide-mémoire (Table 1.1) in more detail.

Follow a protocol

Dimond (1995) and McVey (1996) both stressed the importance of formal protocols for both patient and nurse protection. Even when nurses,

Table 1.1 Safe practice

1. Follow a protocol
2. Accountability (Codes): *Guidelines for the Administration of Medicines* (UKCC 2000), *Code of Professional Conduct* (UKCC 1992a), *The Scope of Professional Practice* (UKCC 1992b)
3. Permission: doctor and nurse management
4. Informed consent – patient or another
5. Competence and qualification
6. Assessment
7. Documentation
8. Evaluation

Having looked at Table 1.1, how would you go about introducing a therapy into your area of practice?
What do you see as being the most difficult hurdles to overcome?

---

employed by the NHS, are qualified in complementary therapies, unless their contract states that these form part of their everyday practice, they cannot use them on patients within their care without express permission from a doctor and senior nurse management (Dimond 1995, McVey 1996). Although as nurses we are constantly encouraged to develop our skills, to do so without the necessary training and consent would be foolish, because such pursuits could not only breach the code of professional conduct (UKCC 1992a), but also negate any vicarious liability of our employer (Stone 1999)! Permission from senior nurse management and the patient's medical consultant must therefore be sought and obtained.

Accountability

Advice about this is provided in the following codes and guidelines: *Guidelines for the Administration of Medicines* (UKCC 2000), *Code of Professional Conduct* (UKCC 1992a) and *The Scope of Professional Practice* (UKCC 1992b). The UKCC states that practice must be safe, recognise the limitations of the practitioner and/or therapy, be aware of any contraindications to practice, work in collaboration with others and be research based. The advice is, however, very limited and somewhat unclear because there are no national guidelines, although Darley (1996) would dispute this as he asserts that the 'Scope' (UKCC 1992b) provides sufficient information to guide safe complementary practice. His article concludes:

The Council believes that its Code of Professional Practice [Conduct] and Scope of Professional Practice offer the type of enabling framework that will allow practitioners registered with the Council to offer complementary therapies to patients safely and responsibly. Consequently patients and clients will be able to benefit from these therapies in a safe, properly sanctioned and appropriate manner.

Darley (1996)

The Royal College of Nursing also provides regular guidance through its *In Touch* newsletter and further expert advice may be obtained from the few policies that have often been devised purely to meet local needs (Pfiel 1994, Wafer 1994). However, McVey (1996) still advises developing policies in relation to *The Scope of Professional Practice* (UKCC 1992a), so that complementary therapies may be incorporated into practice competently. Yet Freshwater (1996) says that this will not be achieved or such practice accepted until care is grounded in research as opposed to 'anec dotal or personal accounts'.

Within the nursing literature, I have found only one account of poor complementary practice that had been reported to the UKCC (Anon 2001a). The article stated that the UKCC had cautioned a male occupational health nurse for offering a patient a personal massage after normal working hours. After offering this, the nurse who also runs a private massage business from home, wrote to the patient requesting him not to mention this to anyone else as he had other allegations pending. It is not, however, clear in this report exactly why he was cautioned.

Permission

Doctor and nurse management (see also 'Protocol' above)

There is potential for conflict here because control over the patient rests mostly with the doctor. Therefore, unless you get permission and support from the doctor concerned, it will be difficult to utilise complementary therapies alongside orthodox care. Remember that providing treatments without medical permission is inherently dangerous.

Managerial consent is also required. Your line manager will act as an agent for your employer and if you practise without their permission tasks that you are not contracted to do you will not be protected by vicarious liability, because your employer could rightly deny any liability. This means that you would be held personally responsible for any harm caused, and if negligence is established you would be legally responsible to pay any compensation due. But if, on the other hand, you can show that you are working within the terms of your employment your employer will endorse you. Of course you still have to abide by your own personal and professional accountability (Stone 1999). Once these decisions have been made, further discussions involving the multi-professional team need to be held to consider the possible implications for practice and also the best way to facilitate this change.

If you are considering using your skills as an independent practitioner within an NHS setting, other rules apply. As such, you have a twofold duty to the patient and would be liable under the laws of negligence and contract of services, e.g. you may not have harmed the patient but may have not done him any good either. If the latter is proved, you will not be found to be negligent but could still be liable for breach of contract (Dimond 1995).

Informed consent

You must always obtain consent from the patient or another, before treatment, and consent should be given to the person undertaking the treatment. If this is not done it may constitute trespass. Although consent need not be in writing, it is preferable to obtain it in this way in case of possible future disputes. The patient must fully understand what is to be done and also be aware that he or she may withdraw from this treatment at any time. Informed consent can be given for a part of or the whole treatment plan (Dimond 1995).

Competence and qualification

Only where standards are set is it possible for any practitioner to determine whether or not they are competent to practise. But how can this be established when most complementary therapies are currently unregulated? Currently the individual therapies of reflexology and aromatherapy are trying to address this issue because national occupational standards (NOS) have been set up in an attempt to set measurable standards that will underpin and provide a common reference point for all future qualifications (Trevelyan 1998b, Baker 2001).

Pre-set standards are important because, in a negligent action, the plaintiff would have to show that the defendant failed to follow standards set and was incompetent (Dimond 1995). Competence can, however, be established by utilising the knowledge and supervision of an approved practitioner, e.g. to ensure that patients receive efficient and competent care it would be necessary for this approved person to set up a teaching programme and involve all who are to practise (McVey 1996). The procedures then need to be practised under supervision and only when deemed competent should they use them with their individual patients. There-fore, with the appropriate permission, as long as you have been taught the skill by a qualified practitioner, even if he or she is not a nurse, you could practise them (Brett 1999). It would, however, be sensible to consider taking out indemnity insurance.

Assessment

Patients must be assessed before any procedure. It is useful to give written as well as verbal information to each patient and their nurses about this. Fully informed consent, before treatment, must be obtained.

Documentation

Consent, treatments, patient experiences and outcomes should be documented in the nursing notes. In addition to this, it is also useful if you record such experiences in your own professional profile.

Evaluation

The primary task is to evaluate the effectiveness of your interventions (Ersser 1995) and adapt them accordingly.

Briefly summarise the steps you would need to take to establish the use of complementary therapies in your practice area.

The integration of complementary therapies into nursing practice is fraught with difficulty and totally dependent on the backing of many others. It is essential that you work collaboratively with others to establish rigorous protocols and procedures, which will sustain you through the ensuing obligatory and inherently complicated change process. In the interests of patient safety, you should seek only to introduce realistic, cost-effective and beneficial therapies, and to make sure that those who will implement them are sufficiently able to do so. Once these are established, it is crucial to evaluate the outcomes and continue to support and encourage others in their future endeavours.

References

Anon (1999) Guidelines for writing proposals for the integration of complementary therapies into clinical nursing practice. In Touch (Newsletter for RCN Complementary Therapies in Nursing Forum) March 6–7.

Anon (2000) Complementary medicine: time for critical engagement. The Lancet **356**: 2023.

Anon (2001a) In brief. Masseur cautioned. Nursing Times **97**(9): 6.

Anon (2001b) Fit for practice: Part 2.4: Scope of professional practice. Nursing Times **97**(8): 47–50.

Baker S (2001) AOC Update. Aromatherapy World: Seeding March 4.

Brett H (1999) Aromatherapy in the care of older people. Nursing Times **95**(33): 56–57.

Brett H, Barker S (1998) Beating the burn. Nursing Times **94**(32): 75–79.

Bell L, Sikora K (1996) Guest editorial. Complementary therapies and cancer care. Complementary Therapies in Nursing and Midwifery **2**: 57–58.

British Medical Association (1986) Alternative Therapy: Report of the Board of Education. London: BMA.

British Medical Association (1993) Complementary Medicine: New approaches to good practice. London: BMA.

Buckle J (1993) When is holism not complementary? British Journal of Nursing **2**: 744–745.

Darley M (1996) Complementary therapies: the position of the UKCC. Complementary Therapies in Nursing and Midwifery **1**: 106–109.

Davis C, ed. (1997) Complementary Therapies in Rehabilitation: Holistic approaches for prevention and wellness. Thorofare, NJ: Slack Inc.

Department of Health (1997) The New NHS: Modern and dependable, Cm 3807. London: DoH.

Dimond B (1995) Legal issues – complementary therapies and the nurse. Complementary Therapies in Nursing and Midwifery **1**: 21–3.

Editorial (2000) The way forward. His Royal Highness The Prince of Wales. Complementary Therapies in Nursing and Midwifery **6**: 1–3.

Eisenberg D, David R, Ettner S et al. (1998) Trends in alternative medicine use in the United States 1990–1997. Journal of the American Medical Association **208**: 1569–1575.

Ernst E, Cassileth B (1998) The prevalence of complementary/alternative medicine in cancer – a systematic review. Cancer **83**: 777–782.

Ernst E, White A (2000) The BBC survey of complementary medicine use in the UK. Complementary Therapies in Medicine **8**: 32–36.

Ersser S (1995) Complementary therapies and nursing research: issues and practicalities. Complementary Therapies in Nursing and Midwifery **1**: 44–45.

European Commission (1998) COST Action B4. Unconventional medicine: final report of the Management Committee 1993–98.

Foundation for Integrated Medicine (1997) Integrated Health Care: A way forward for the next five years. London: FIM.

Freshwater D (1996) Complementary therapies and research in nursing practice. Nursing Standard **10**(38): 43–45.

Fulder S (1988) Cited in Sidell (1995).

Gennis F (1992) Alternative roads to hell? Nursing Standard **6**(44): 42–43.

Good M (1995) Relaxation techniques for surgical patients. American Journal of Nursing **5**: 39–43.

Goodman H (1995) Patients' views count as well. Nursing Standard **9**(40): 55.

HAS (1997) Services for People who are Elderly: Addressing the balance. London: The Stationery Office.

HAS (1998) Not Because They Are Old: An independent enquiry into the care of older people on acute wards in general hospitals. London: Health Advisory Service.

Henwood M (1992) Through a Glass Darkly: Community care and elderly people. King's Fund Institute Project 14. London: King's Fund Centre.

Kendrick K (1999) Challenging power, autonomy and politics in complementary therapies: a contentious view. Complementary Therapies in Nursing and Midwifery 5: 77–81.

Kiddel M (1986) The meaning of illness. Holistic Medicine 1: 15–26.

Long A, Mercer G, Hughes K (2000) developing a tool to measure holistic practice: a missing dimension in outcome measurement with complementary therapies. Complementary Therapies in Medicine 8: 26–31.

McVey M (1996) Practice. Policy development. Complementary Therapies in Nursing and Midwifery 2: 41–46.

Montbriand M (1991) Alternative health care as a control strategy. Journal of Advanced Nursing 16: 325–332.

Naish J (1997) Nursing and the law. Danger zones. Nursing Times 93(16): 24–26.

National Association of Health Authorities and Trusts (1993) Complementary Therapies in the NHS (Research Paper No. 10). London: National Association of Health Authorities and Trusts.

News (1996) WHO warns of nurse shortages. Nursing Times 92(24): 9.

Peace G, Simmons D (1996) Completing the whole. Nursing Times 92(25): 52–54.

Pfiel M (1994) Role of nurses in promoting complementary therapies. British Journal of Nursing 3: 217–219.

Pietroni P (1992) Beyond the boundaries: relationship between general practice and complementary medicine. British Medical Journal 305: 564–566.

Rankin-Box D (1991) Proceed with caution. Nursing Times 87(45): 34–36.

Rankin-Box D (1997) Therapies in practice: a survey assessing nurses' use of complementary therapies. Complementary Therapies in Nursing and Midwifery 3: 92–9.

Royal Commission on Long Term Care (1999) With Respect to Old Age: A report by the Royal Commission on long term care, CM 4192-1. London: Stationery Office.

Sidell M (1995) Rethinking Ageing: Health in old age, myth, mystery and management. Buckingham: Open University Press.

Stevensen C (1994) The psychophysical effects of aromatherapy massage following cardiac surgery. Complementary Therapies in Nursing and Midwifery 2: 27–35.

Stone J (1999) Using complementary therapies within nursing: some ethical and legal considerations. Complementary Therapies in Nursing and Midwifery 5: 46–50.

Sutcliffe A (2001) Complementary therapies and Christianity. Aromatherapy World March 28–30.

Trevelyan J (1998a) Complementary therapies on the NHS: current practice, future development (Part 1). Complementary Therapies in Nursing and Midwifery 4: 82–84.

Trevelyan J (1998b) Future of complementary medicine: training, status and the European perspective (Part 2). Complementary Therapies in Nursing and Midwifery 4: 108–110.

United Kingdom Central Council for Nursing, Midwifery and Health Visiting (1992a) Code of Professional Conduct. London: UKCC.

United Kingdom Central Council for Nursing, Midwifery and Health Visiting (1992b) The Scope of Professional Practice. London: UKCC.

United Kingdom Central Council for Nursing, Midwifery and Health Visiting (2000) Guidelines for the Administration of Medicines. London: UKCC.

Wafer M (1994) Finding the formula to enhance care: Guideline for the use of complementary therapies in nursing practice. Professional Nurse March: 414–417.

World Health Report (1997) Conquering Suffering Enriching Humanity. Geneva: World Health Organization.

Wright S (1995) Bringing the heart back into nursing. Complementary Therapies in Nursing and Midwifery 1: 15–20.

CHAPTER 2

The appropriateness of touch

Although there is a huge amount written about touch, the aim of this chapter is to provide only a very brief introduction to what it constitutes and also the implications of using it! Historically various types of touch have been used for healing and the comfort of patients. Touch is one of the first senses to develop and is said to be integral to effective verbal and non-verbal communication. Although touch is often regarded as a universal language, it appears that our perceptions of it are very much influenced by our formative years. It would seem therefore that the ability to appreciate and respond positively to touch in later years is dependent on our experience of touch during infancy (Simms 1994).

Watson (1975) defined touch as:

> . . . an intentional physical contact between two or more individuals . . .

and went on to divide it into two separate categories. He described one as instrumental (or that used in our everyday nursing procedures) and the other as expressive, which he said was a more spontaneous and affectionate type of touch.

The use and acceptance of touch appear to be dependent on social and cultural norms and mores. Argyle (1978) stated that there are both contact and non-contact cultures within the world. The former tend to be from places such as northern Africa, whereas the latter tend to be mostly from much of Europe, including Britain, and North America. It patently holds very different meanings for different cultures, e.g. within the Hindu caste system, it would be totally inappropriate to touch someone from the lowest 'sudras' caste because to do so would result in contamination and necessitate a rigorous cleansing regimen to be instigated (Montague 1971). We may need to consider this more now that the world has become a 'global village', especially as we all tend to live and work within such multicultural communities.

The British are said to be particularly undemonstrative and less emotional than other races and also very keen to maintain their personal space. This has been seen as an inherent protective mechanism to prevent over-familiarisation and personal 'invasion'. Barnett (1972) identified this need for personal space and also stressed that on some occasions, because of this, touch might actually be contraindicated.

Touch is also influenced by gender. When reviewing studies that had looked at gender and touch, Stier and Hall (1984) concluded that females initiated touch more than males, there was some tendency for them to receive more touch than males, and also that females touched other females more than males touched other males. Touch is sometimes associated with sex, so that touching someone can be open to misinterpretation. It is essential to consider the appropriateness of your actions, because touch may be acceptable only under clearly defined circumstances (Le May 1986). Touch is not always used nicely because it may be used to inflict deliberate harm on another. For some, then, it is associated only with violence and abusive situations.

The role of touch

It would seem that nurses require educating in the subtleties of touch. It is therefore imperative for you to be able to identify the type, amount and extent of touch that any of your individual patients could comfortably tolerate. Remember that touch will be experienced differently by everybody, felt differently in different parts of the body, and may be received passively, actively or as therapy. But touch can be used very simply, for instance, when we pat or gently touch another it may merely convey comfort, reassurance and support.

Simms (1994) recalled the effect that touch had on one of her newly widowed patients during her first night in an acute admission ward of a psychiatric hospital. The patient said:

> I remember feeling very lonely, sad and distressed. I was overwhelmed with confusion and fear . . . . I cannot remember if I actually called out for help, but the night nurse came and just held my hand. I shall never forget the warmth and acceptance of that touch – during that dreadful night!

Simms (1994)

Types of touch

Tutton (1991), when defining the type of touch used in nursing, built very much on Watson's (1975) concepts and added a further two categories (see 3 and 4 below). They are summarised below:

1. Instrumental touch: this is the type of mechanical touch used most often by nurses in their everyday practice, because it is associated with 'doing necessary things' for patients, such as performing a blanket bath, taking a temperature, etc.
2. Expressive touch: this constitutes activities, such as cuddling a patient or perhaps holding their hand reassuringly, while they are experiencing a painful procedure or grieving over a loved one.
3. Systematic touch: this would be where a set manipulative therapy, e.g. massage or reflexology, is used in the planned treatment of patients.
4. Therapeutic touch (TT): this is almost a misnomer because here patients experience a form of healing touch that does not involve the nurse touching their actual physical body. Instead the aura or magnetic field surrounding the patient's body is contacted.

Routasalo (1996), however, used a very different kind of terminology when she stated that within nursing care there were two kinds of touch. Interestingly she labelled them necessary and non-necessary touch (NNT)! Her study found that most patients received necessary touch (that given during the performance of a nursing task) and also that nurses used NNT quite often, but predominantly with their 'favourite' patients and with the aim of 'making their message personal'. It would seem that, although she chose such an emotive term for this type of touch, she was, like other researchers, looking to see how much expressive touch patients received, and not as the descriptor implies, receiving touch when they should not!

The appropriateness of touch

Although the benefits of touch are well documented and touching patients is a part of every nurse's daily activity, some patients find it threatening (Vortherms 1991). As has already been stated, the enjoyment of being touched is influenced by individual cultural norms and taboos, and also by personal upbringing. One must remember that many of the older people who are now being cared for were often taught to adopt a somewhat reticent manner, 'the stiff upper lip' code of behaviour, so it is appropriate to consider these issues before embarking on activities that would violate this.

Horrigan (1995) said that:

> British people have a reputation for being reserved – touch is considered a private and intimate activity, often linked with sex.

Sometimes to touch is quite inappropriate, would be considered invasive and may even harm the patient–nurse relationship. But nurses also have rights and they must also feel comfortable about touching. Any genuine concerns about this should be recognised because touching another inevitably involves risks.

Autton (1996), a former hospital chaplain, when recounting his personal experiences with dying patients, noted that, although using empathetic touch with some individuals permitted them, at this time, to 'open up' more readily and unburden their innermost fears and worries, the timing was crucial. He felt that if you got this wrong, patients would actually 'clam up' and the special moment would be lost. He also felt very strongly that sometimes it was better not to touch so that you did not give out the wrong signals to these vulnerable patients. He recognised, however, that it was difficult to judge this accurately, especially if you had not been in the fortunate position of being able to build up a special rapport with these patients.

Tobiason (1986) asserted that, as people aged, their need for touch increased, but events in their lives may inhibit this from being a reality. As a result of bereavement and isolation, etc., the opportunities for this may be far less than in earlier life. Watson (1975) found that older dependent people are often deprived of expressive touch. Burnside (1973) also found that nurses tended to restrict the use of touch with these older individuals. This is so sad because he noted how such touch could often reduce sensory deprivation in them as a result of its intrinsic value in non-verbal communication. It was also felt that intimate touch might partly compensate them for their losses associated with bereavement, dependency and even altered body image.

Autton (1996) observed how not only carers, but also relatives, tended to withdraw from intimate contact the nearer to death a patient became and he wrote:

> Visitors, including relatives, often withdraw from the bedside and so leave the patient not only mentally and emotionally, but physically isolated as well. The kiss on the lips becomes a peck on the forehead, then the light touch on the arm, then the wave from the door. When the doctor visits, he stands at the foot of the bed.
>
> Autton (1996)

I think all of us can relate to such an emotive statement!

Touch within health care

Pratt and Mason (1984) stated that there had been little research into the significance of touch in health care, but asserted that all health professionals, by virtue of their occupation, had been allowed to access any patient's personal space or body freely. As a result of this freedom they have more opportunity than most to touch people. But because of the unequal power base inherent within carer and client relationships, it may sometimes be used inappropriately and wrongly. And, although it is not within the remit of this chapter to define and discuss the controversial theories surrounding practitioner–client abuse, I feel that it is necessary to interject a word of caution.

Lipley (1999) notes how the United Kingdom Central Council (UKCC) has had to develop guidelines about this. This document, *Practitioner–Client Relationships and the Prevention of Abuse*, was sent to all nurses, midwives and heath visitors at the end of 1999, and their message is clearly one of 'zero tolerance'. He cites part of the evidence given by one of the victims at the misconduct trial of a community psychiatric nurse (CPN):

> When my husband died, I went to see a spiritualist who told me that my husband would send someone to help me and look after me.

All of us will be ashamed to read that, instead of this someone helping her (not the spiritualist), over 6 years the CPN managed to have sex with her and also to extort from her over £25 000! This was discovered only after she had attempted suicide twice. He was struck off. Lipley (1999) also states that the Royal College of Nursing (RCN) firmly support these measures and have applauded the UKCC for having the courage to develop them. The RCN do, however, remind us that the vast majority of nurses provide 'effective and appropriate care'.

Once recognised, it is relatively easy to deal with such a straightforward case of abuse, but difficulties arise where there are 'grey areas' of practice to investigate, because the true intention behind any nurse's touch cannot always be assumed. Although not being alarmist, it is imperative that nurses are aware that they may, at times, walk a very fine line between what is perfectly acceptable for them to do and what may be deliberately or accidentally misconstrued by either party involved. This is never more so than when practising the touch therapies.

Touch therapies and their use

One small-scale study by McCann and McKenna (1993) examined the amount and type of touch that their elderly institutionalised patients were receiving. While recognising that these small-scale findings were not readily generalisable across all elderly populations, they did feel that some of their findings were very pertinent.

The results suggested that:

- most of the touch (95.3%) was of the instrumental type
- most instrumental touch and all expressive touch was to the extremities (expressive touching of the trunk was not observed)
- the patients interviewed appeared to feel comfortable with instrumental touch but were not so comfortable with facial or upper leg contact.

They therefore concluded that patients could easily misconstrue more intimate forms of touch. As a result of this they recommended that because not all the patients were receptive to touch nurses should be aware of this and be extra sensitive to the verbal and non-verbal cues that a patient may give out about this.

Sanderson and Carter (1994) felt that touch therapies gave patients not only the opportunity to develop good relationships with their therapists, but also to make them feel that they were the prime focus of care. But practising tactile therapies may give nurses another medium in which they may be able to express greater caring and sensitivity. There is some evidence that nurses are becoming disenchanted with their increasingly technical role and, although they are often highly educated and qualified, they are mourning the loss of some of their traditional 'nursing' skills. They appear then not only to be taking them on for the benefit of their patients, but perhaps also seeking different avenues to fulfil themselves. It has been suggested that, by taking on more of these therapies, they may be able to return to the 'heart of nursing' (Wright 1995)!

This is not a very new idea because the Commission on Nursing, or Briggs Report as it is commonly referred to, recorded back in 1972 that increasing numbers of nurses were adopting modalities that might enable them to 'escape the production line concept of care' (Wright 1995). Patients appear also to be disappointed with nurses and other healthcare personnel's seeming obsession with technical tasks and are said to feel isolated and even debased by these activities. Older's (1982) observation may sum up this feeling. He noticed that even patient examination had become more technical and impersonal and asked whether:

. . . human contact is always mediated through the steel of the stethoscope, the wood
of the tongue depressor, or the rubber of the patella hammer?

Older (1982)

This might be too simplistic an example, but he was merely intimating
that we do not use our hands very much with patients these days. One
returning nurse, after her second shift, remarked to me that she had been
on duty for more than 8 hours and had never once touched a patient. I do
not know how unusual this is, but you might like to think when you are next
on duty just how many times you touch a patient in the course of a shift!

Healing and healers

There have been healers around for many centuries, but unfortunately
their work has often been associated with black magic and the work of the
devil. Although healing appears to be more acceptable in the UK than in
other parts of the Western World, it still suffers from misunderstanding
and cynicism. Benor (1991) noted that, although there was considerable
anecdotal, clinical and experimental research-based evidence to support
its efficacy, many doctors and scientists still would rather believe that
healing just exerted a placebo reaction in its gullible recipient and that it
was normally offered by charlatans. This thinking has probably arisen
because healing is often associated, in some people's minds, with 'miracle
cures', faith healing and spiritualism. Yet modern-day healers are very
well regulated and mostly belong to associations that set standards and
codes of conduct for their members.

Healing involves the 'laying on of hands' and although some practitioners believe that their powers of healing are 'channelled' through them,
by some divine entity, others do not. It is felt, however, that there is some
exchange of 'energy' between the healer and the recipient (Benor 1991).
Although healing might seem to be rather mystical and different from how
we practise nursing, one study revealed that nurses and healers often
shared a common holistic philosophy. As a result of this, Engebretson
(1996) felt that nurses were ideally placed to help those in orthodox care to
appreciate why patients sought alternative techniques and also could help
legitimise them.

One therapy where this seems to have happened is therapeutic touch
(TT), because it was developed by a nurse, Dolores Krieger, and a
renowned healer, Dora Kunz. A literature search revealed a vast amount of
literature on TT, but it is not possible, within the confines of this chapter or
the author's experience, to be able to review it all. It included the following:

- a discussion on its conceptual basis and procedural issues (Heidt 1991, Booth 1993, McCormack and Galantino 1997, Mackereth and Wright 1997)
- research-based studies and reviews (Benor 1991, Wirth et al. 1993)
- the experiences of patients and practitioners, some of which are written as experimental case studies, whereas others are purely subjective and anecdotal accounts (Heidt 1991, Green 1996a, 1996b, Mills 1996, Hayes and Cox 1999).

On the whole, I found that most of what is written appeared to extol its benefits and strove to provide evidence to support its continued use.

One small study (Rosa et al. 1998), the first of its kind, provided a dissenting voice when it sought to question whether TT practitioners really could perceive the 'human energy field' (HEF). Over several months, practitioners were asked to detect a researcher's hand, which was shielded from them by a screen. It was hypothesised that, because TT works by detecting the HEF, the practitioners should be able to detect the researcher's hand every time. Unfortunately the results revealed a success rate of only 44%. It was therefore concluded that this proved that the claims of TT were groundless and that its further use was unjustified.

TT does, however, appear to be a somewhat confusing term because people often refer to using touch with patients meaningfully as therapeutic touch. It would perhaps be better, when referring to this, to say the therapeutic use of touch so that the therapy TT can more readily be identified. It seems almost to be misnamed because only the aura and not the physical body is touched, although some practitioners do employ touch, as well, during the treatment sessions.

The development of TT

Therapeutic touch appears to have developed out of the work of several people. Grad, a Canadian biologist concluded after studying healing, that it was not suggestion that influenced healing but a transfer of some kind of energy. Even today it is still not known exactly what this energy is. Some say that to perform this therapy you do not need to be formally trained in it, but modern-day TT practitioners may dispute this.

At much the same time, Martha Rogers was working on her complex model (1970), in which she identified that humans did not have energy fields but were energy fields. She also theorised that there is a continual and mutual exchange of energy between all parts of the universe (Booth 1993). This is summed up in the following comprehensive definition of nursing, which for the 1970s, must have been very far reaching indeed. She asserted that:

> Nursing aims to assist people in achieving their maximum health potential. Nursing is concerned with people – all people – well and sick, rich and poor, young and old. The arenas of nursing's services extend into all areas where there are people – on this planet and now moving into outer space. Nursing's body of scientific knowledge is a new product specific to nursing. Concomitantly the science of nursing does not arise out of a vacuum, nor [is it] necessarily, of meaning only to nurses. Nursing is a humanistic science.
>
> Rogers (1970)

Similarly, Dolores Krieger and Dora Kunz began to investigate and promote methods in which the body could use its own latent energy for the purpose of self-healing. Their work appears to be built on the same assumptions as those expressed by Rogers (1970). Krieger's theory sought to marry the best from healing with the best from traditional nursing practice (Simms 1994). But it seems that she primarily, developed this therapy in the 1960s, within the USA, because of her dissatisfaction with the then current nursing system.

Many authors use Meehan's (1990) definition, presented below, to describe TT and its practice:

> A knowledgeable and purposive patterning of patient–environmental energy field process in which the nurse assumes a meditative form of awareness and uses her hands as a focus for the patterning of the mutual patient–environmental energy field process.
>
> Meehan (1990)

But, this seems to be a hugely complicated set of words that need unravelling. Booth (1993) describes it much more simply as:

> . . . a technique based on an idea that there is a universal energy flow and all living organisms are part of its field.
>
> Booth (1993)

He goes on to explain that any disturbance of an individual's energy field will result in illness. This imbalance can be ameliorated by the TT practitioner if he or she can repattern (rebalance) their energy field. This is said to be accomplished only if the energy fields of the therapist and patient interact.

TT procedure

Booth (1993) states that most writers on TT identify the following sequence:

1. Centring (or centering) – here the practitioner prepares to treat the patient.
2. Assessment – the practitioner runs his or her hands around the aura of the patient's body, trying to pick up (feel) any clues about the patient's condition.
3. Clearing – the practitioner's hands sweep the aura of the body in an attempt to aid the energy flow.
4. Intervention – here an attempt is made to rebalance the patient's energy.
5. Evaluation – here the practitioner decides when the treatment is complete.

McCormack and Galantino (1997) state that two conditions must be present before TT, or NCTT (non-contact therapeutic touch) as they term it, may be practised effectively. They are:

• Intentionality – before treating anyone practitioners must clear their minds so that they are 'open' to the healing needs of the recipient.
• Assessment – practitioners must sweep their hands over the recipient's body about 3–6 inches (7–15 cm) away, so that they can detect any imbalances or 'other perceivable sensations'.

The treatment should take about 20 minutes and the patient should be allowed some time to rest afterwards. An evaluation of the procedure should be attempted, and subjective and objective observations recorded. Some practitioners record their findings pictorially on anatomical charts as well as writing traditional notes. A plan should be made for the next intervention.

Although TT has been introduced into Great Britain only fairly recently and is still in its infancy, Lewis (1999) feels that because of growing interest in TT and the number of practitioners qualifying, within the country 'the profile of TT is set to rise' (see Further reading for informative texts on TT).

It is inevitable that touch will play an integral part in the following touch therapies presented in this book. As elderly patients can feel deprived of physical contact and therefore socially isolated in times of stress, you may need to seek ways with which to bring more holistic care to them (Vortherms 1991). But remember that there are taboos associated with culture, sex and often with different parts of the body, which must be considered. Watson (1975) in his subjective study reported that, the greater the amount of expressive touch given, the further it is (normally) given away from the taboo areas of the body! This parameter is likely to change when practising some of the tactile therapies.

Your traditional role as a nurse has given you freedom of access to patients, and although you have performed intimate care for them many times, participating in complementary therapies will be seen in a different context. This may be as much to do with the controversies and power struggles surrounding them, as the differences in care that you will perform. Perhaps before you embark on the process of learning how to utilise touch appropriately and effectively within the boundaries of the touch therapies, you could contemplate the following:

> Nursing, real nursing is not so much about what nurses do but the way they do it. The application of the knowledge base, the touching, teaching, observing, comforting
> . . . being with expressive skills, give nurses that crucial role for patients, of humanizing health care and making it therapeutic.
>
> Pearson (1988)

Questions

Try to answer the following:

1. Identify some of the types of touch and the appropriateness of their use.
2. What is the difference between using touch therapeutically and the therapy therapeutic touch (TT)?
3. How was therapeutic touch developed and who were influential in its promotion?
4. Discuss some of the taboos associated with touch.
5. Can you identify some of the more common touch therapies that nurses are keen to use with older patients?

References

Argyle M (1978) The Psychology of Interpersonal Behaviour. Harmondsworth: Penguin.

Autton N (1996) The use of touch in palliative care. European Journal of Palliative Care 3(3): 121.

Barnett K (1972) A theoretical construction of the concepts of touch as they relate to nursing. Nursing Research 21: 102–110.

Benor D (1991) Spiritual healing in clinical practice. Nursing Times 87(44): 35–37.

Booth B (1993) Therapeutic touch. Nursing Times 89(31): 48–50.

Burnside I (1973) Touching is talking. American Journal of Nursing 73: 2060–2063.

Engebretson J (1996) Comparison of nurses and alternative healers. IMAGE: Journal of Nursing Scholarship 28: 959.

Green C (1996a) A reflection of a Therapeutic Touch experience: Case study 1. Complementary Therapies in Nursing and Midwifery 2: 122–125.

Green C (1996b) Reflection of a Therapeutic Touch experience: Case study 2. Complementary Therapies in Nursing and Midwifery 4: 17–21.

Hayes J, Cox C (1999) The experience of therapeutic touch from a nursing perspective. British Journal of Nursing 8: 1249–1254.

Heidt P (1991) Helping patients to rest: Clinical studies in therapeutic touch. Holistic Nursing Practice 5(4): 57–66.

Horrigan C (1995) Massage. In: Rankin-Box D, ed., The Nurses' Handbook of Complementary Therapies. Edinburgh: Churchill Livingstone.

Le May A (1986) The human connection. Nursing Times 82(47:) 28–30.

Lewis D (1999) A survey of therapeutic touch practitioners. Nursing Standard 13(30): 33–37.

Lipley N (1999) Analysis. Close encounters. Nursing Standard 14(3): 10.

McCann K, McKenna H (1993) An examination of touch between nurses and elderly patients in a continuing care setting in Northern Ireland. Journal of Advanced Nursing 18: 030–846.

McCormack G, Galantino M (1997) Non-contact therapeutic touch. In: Davis C, ed. Complementary Therapies in Rehabilitation: Holistic approaches for prevention and wellness. Thorofare, NJ: Slack Inc.

Mackereth P, Wright J (1997) Therapeutic touch: nursing activity or form of spiritual healing? Complementary Therapies in Nursing and Midwifery 3: 106–110.

Meehan T (1990) Theory development. In: Barrett E, ed., Visions of Rogers' Science-based Nursing. New York: National League for Nursing.

Mills A (1996) Therapeutic Touch – case study: The application, documentation and outcome. Complementary Therapies in Medicine 4: 127–132.

Montague M (1971) The Human Significance of Skin. New York: Columbia University Press.

Older J (1982) Touch is Healing. New York: Stein & Day.

Pearson A (1988) Trends in Clinical Nursing. London: Croom Helm.

Pratt J, Mason A (1984) The meaning of touch in care practice. Social Science and Medicine 18: 1081–1088.

Rogers M (1970) An Introduction to the Theoretical Basis of Nursing. PA: FA Davis Co.

Rosa L, Rosa E, Sarner L, Barrett S (1998) A close look at therapeutic touch. Journal of the American Medical Association 279: 1005–1010.

Routasalo P (1996) Non-necessary touch in the nursing care of elderly people. Journal of Advanced Nursing 25: 904–911.

Sanderson H, Carter A (1994) Healing hands – aromatherapy – helping patients with learning disabilities to relax. Nursing Times 90(11): 46–48.

Simms J (1994) Alternative therapies. In: Wright H, Giddey M, eds, Mental Health Nursing. From first principles to professional practice. London: Chapman & Hall.

Stier D, Hall J (1984) gender differences in touch: an empirical and theoretical revue. Journal of Personality and Social Psychology 47: 440–449.

Tobiason S (1986) Touching is for everyone. American Journal of Nursing 4: 78–80.

Tutton L (1991) An exploration of touch and its use in nursing. In: McMahon R, Pearson A, eds, Nursing as a Therapy. London: Chapman & Hall, pp 142–169.

Vortherms R (1991) Clinically improving communication through touch. Journal of Gerontological Nursing 17: 5.

Watson W (1975) The meaning of touch: geriatric nursing. Journal of Communication 25(3): 104–112.

Wirth D, Richardson J, Eidelman W, O'Malley A (1993) Full thickness dermal wounds treated with non contact Therapeutic Touch: a replication and extension. Complementary Therapies in Medicine 1: 127–32.

Wright S (1995) Bringing the heart back into nursing. Complementary Therapies in Nursing and Midwifery 1: 15–20.

Further reading

Keller E, Bzdek V (1986) Effects of therapeutic touch on tension headache pain. Nursing Research 35: 102–106.

Mills A, Biley F (1994) A case study in Rogerian Nursing. Nursing Standard 9(7): 31–34.

Olsen M, Sneed N (1995) Anxiety and therapeutic touch. Issues in Mental Health Nursing 16: 97–108.

Sayre-Adams J (1992) Therapeutic touch, research and reality. Nursing Standard 2(50): 52–54.

Sayre-Adams J (1993) Therapeutic Touch – principles and practice. Complementary Therapies in Medicine 1: 96–99.

Sayre-Adams J (1995) Theory and Practice of Therapeutic Touch. Edinburgh: Churchill Livingstone.

Watson W (1975) The meanings of touch: geriatric nursing. Journal of Communication 25: 104–112.

PART II

An overview of therapies

An increasingly wide range of therapies are now being used by nurses across the UK and this section will introduce you to four therapies that are among those most commonly used by them. Undoubtedly there has been an escalation in their popularity and Stevensen (1997, page 50) questions whether this:

> ... selection of predominantly hands-on therapies [merely reflects] nurses' desire to reinforce the caring role which they are striving to keep, given the demands on their time in other aspects of their work.
>
> Stevensen (1997)

In this second part, although it is not intended to be a definitive guide to the following therapies, it will give you an opportunity to look at their historical influences, theoretical underpinnings and practical application, and contemplate how accurate Stevensen's (1997) assumption might be!

Reference

Stevensen C (1997) Complementary therapies and their role in nursing care. Nursing Standard 11(24), 49–55.

CHAPTER 3

Massage

Massage involves the manipulation of soft tissues for therapeutic purposes and may be performed on most parts of the body utilising a variety of techniques, all involving different degrees of pressure. Depending on the individual patient's need, it may be used either in a gentle and soothing way to induce relaxation or more vigorously to stimulate them. Massage is very effective in painful and chronic conditions such as arthritis, stroke and multiple sclerosis, especially where immobility is a problem, and may be used alone or in conjunction with essential oils (this is explained in Chapter 4). Although many advocate that to benefit from treatment patients need to experience a whole body massage, in my experience they do not. Indeed, in present healthcare settings, you would not necessarily have either the time or the resources to do this. It may therefore be better: carefully to caress a paralysed stroke patient's hand, gently to effleurage a sore knee, shoulder or hip, to manipulate tense neck muscles and to soothe a furrowed brow rather than not offer anything at all. Massage by its very nature is a tactile therapy and, although it has been highlighted that it is particularly desirable for older patients to be touched more, you must be aware that your patients may be wary of experiencing it in this way. This may be influenced further by their cultural and ethical beliefs and even by their gender.

Aim

The word massage appears to be derived from many languages and although it is generally believed to have come from the Arabic 'mass' or 'Mas'h' which means to press softly, it is also associated with the French, Greek and Hindi languages for shampooing and pressing. As this suggests, massage aims to use specific manual techniques to rebalance and strengthen affected areas of the body in order to create and maintain the best possible health for the individual. It also attempts to relax and/or stimulate the mind and body and builds on the power of touch. One only has to witness how someone in pain will, almost without thinking, stroke or rub the affected part of their body in order to ease and aid healing.

Perhaps because of some of the words used above to explain massage techniques, its practice may, unfortunately in some quarters, including the media, still be deliberately misinterpreted as a sexual rather than a therapeutic procedure. You therefore need to be very aware of the language you use to explain it, so that you do not create unnecessary alarm among your patients.

Massage and the ageing skin

Even though studies have tried to identify how massage works it is still not totally clear, although theories have suggested that during massage of the soft tissues and muscles knotted tissues are broken down and immobile joints are freed. This causes potential toxins to be released into the system which are then eliminated from the body via the lymphatic and blood circulations. This may have implications for an older person because age-related changes might affect the integrity of their skin. As ageing takes place the structure of the skin alters. The dermal layer flattens because of a loss of papillae and this, in turn, makes the attachment between the dermis and epidermis less stable. The skin of an older person is often dry, thin and wrinkled, and, although the precise cause of wrinkles is not totally understood, it is thought to result partly from a loss of elastic and subcutaneous fatty tissue, which may be influenced by the collagen and elastin changes in the dermis. The dryness is a result of atrophy of the sebaceous and sweat glands which are then thought to secrete less moisture.

Throughout the skin there are also a large number of nerve endings that are sensitive to temperature, pain, touch and pressure, and some of these nerve endings are affected by age. During massage, it is thought that, as the skin is a very sensitive organ, if the sensory receptors are stimulated they are likely to interact with the rest of the nervous system and in some circumstances may be able to inhibit the pain receptors in the skin and thus reduce pain. In the older person, however, local sensations are often diminished and this may cause the natural and protective reflexes of the skin to be less responsive to harmful situations. Although there is considerable variation among ageing individuals and changes in their skin, tactile sensitivity definitely diminishes. In very old people, however, sensitivity to pain seems to increase again and it is thought that because of excessive thinning of the skin more nerve endings are exposed.

In addition to the above, external and exposed areas of the skin often become pigmented, and fingernails and toenails tend to thicken and become brittle. The progressive degeneration of small blood vessels and capillaries, even in protected skin, is a consequence of ageing that restricts the amount of fluids available to nourish the skin. It is thought that this may also cause drying, thinning and greying of the hair.

As a result of these physiological changes associated with normal ageing, it is vital to consider the following before massaging an older person:

- Because of the reduced blood supply any wounds are likely to heal more slowly and become more easily infected.
- Body temperature regulation is less efficient because of reduced dilatation and contractability of the superficial blood vessels.
- Poor moving of these patients will put them further at risk of skin damage because the ageing skin's epidermis will shear off more easily.
- As older skin is often dry, it is imperative that you differentiate between that and dehydrated skin because it will require extra care.
- Where oedema, either localised and temporary or more widespread, is present, it should be investigated to preclude serious illness. Once a satisfactory medical diagnosis has been made massage can be initiated. Oedema is responsive to massage, but extra care is required if the tissues feel 'soggy' because such skin is very easily damaged.

A brief history of the development of massage

Massage is probably one of the oldest known ways of healing and there is evidence that the Chinese were using this form of therapy at least 3000 years before the birth of Christ. The *Yellow Emperor's Inner Classic (Huangdi Neijing)* is one of the earliest and most influential Chinese medical textbooks, and was written around 300 BC; it contains the earliest Chinese references to massage. Schools of traditional Chinese medicine still use it as a source of information today. The ancient Japanese and Indian societies also had forms of massage around this time and books describing Ayurvedic practices, written slightly later, recommended rubbing and shampooing to help self-healing. The Bible and Qur'an also contain examples of the 'laying on of hands'.

Other references to the efficacy and curative powers of massage for particular conditions are contained in Egyptian, Persian and Japanese texts. The Romans and Greeks were also supporters of the therapeutic effects of massage. Within Homer's *Odyssey* there are descriptions of rubbing exhausted soldiers with oil after battle, and Galen was noted for using massage on the gladiators of Pergamum, pre- and post-tournaments. Many of these ideas have influenced current sports medicine. In addition Hippocrates, the father of medicine, believed that all physicians should be trained in the massaging of stiff joints, but also identified when it was unwise to massage, and is said to have written in the fifth century BC that 'massage reduces fat, strengthens the muscles and firms the skin'. Further evidence is also recorded in the writings of Plato and Socrates, and it is reported that Julius Caesar, who suffered from a form of neuralgia, and Pliny, the Roman naturalist who suffered from recurring bouts of asthma, were both helped by a daily massage.

The popularity of massage began to decline during the Middle Ages as the upsurge in Christianity tended to encourage the view that anything related to physical bodily pleasures was sinful. It was not until the Renaissance that interest in the body and physical health became acceptable and popular once again. Two influential physicians – Abmbroise Paré (AD 1517–1590), a physician to the King of France, and Mercurialis (AD 1530–1606), the attending physician to Mary Queen of Scots – both began to integrate massage extensively into their medical practices.

The development of modern day massage is often attributed to Per Henrik Ling (1776–1839), but Goldstone (2000) disputes this. He felt that there were many other physicians before and after Ling who contributed to the wealth of information now available on massage. He asserts that it is Mezgar, the Dutch physician, rather than Per Ling, the movement therapist, who should be credited with the introduction of modern massage. Even so, Ling was a huge proponent of the art of gymnastics and studied it for many years and out of these studies he developed an exercise programme that was practised in Swedish schools and their armed forces for many years. From this he further developed the 'Swedish System' or 'Lingism' which combined therapeutic massage with exercises for muscles and joints. But this only became known as Swedish massage when it was used abroad.

Goldstone (2000) noted that currently massage seems to belong solely to unorthodox practitioners, yet even as late as the nineteenth and first half of the twentieth centuries it was the province of both medical practitioners and nurses. He also added that, when recounting the history of massage, the 'classical' literature, written at this time, supporting massage as an orthodox treatment is virtually ignored. He added that there were various texts written solely for nurses and also examples of nurses being taught massage, by doctors, in famous hospitals such as St Thomas' and the Royal Orthopaedic Hospital at Stanmore. Such instruction gave advice about not only massage procedures but also how to apply them to specific medical and orthopaedic conditions. The benefits of massage therapy seems to have been appreciated at that time and Hughes (1907) wrote:

> A certificate in massage is held to be an almost essential qualification for a fully qualified nurse to possess.
>
> Cited in Goldstone (2000)

Undoubtedly, however, massage did begin to decline as an orthodox therapy by the 1930s and this appears to have escalated even more with the advent of post-war developments in physiotherapy and the formidable expense involved when providing such a labour-intensive service. Goldstone (2000) asserts, therefore, that massage is not a new complementary therapy but just an orthodox practice that has been re-introduced, albeit in a less standardised and imprecise style.

The advantages and therapeutic benefits of massage

Massage appears to benefit most of the systems of the body, both physically and emotionally. It has been said that the function of every internal organ can be improved, directly or indirectly, by the application of the many different techniques and, although many claims are made about this, some are inevitably anecdotal and excessive. Critics say that, although there have been a few research studies conducted, there is a dearth of good quality research about either the mechanics or efficacy of massage therapy. Vickers (1996) asserts that the available research is often very small scale, sometimes flawed and often too anecdotal. He feels that before this therapy is adopted wholeheartedly it needs further and much more rigorous research to support the claims.

Nurses are now beginning to take up the challenge of providing good quality supporting evidence for their massage practice. There is a need to do this because most of the earlier research was undertaken by non-nurses. Although Hobbs and Davies (1998) feel that nurses must 'grasp the nettle' and evaluate this therapy in order to maintain patient safety and promote clinical effectiveness, they noted that when they tried to research it they encountered methodological difficulties, especially when trying actually to measure what occurred between the patient and the therapist. They are currently developing tools to address such methodological constraints. Although not discounting the value of researching practice, because of the unique experiences of patients, it may be inevitable that some of the 'evidence' gleaned from both patients and nurses/practitioners may be somewhat anecdotal!

The benefits and advantages may include the following:

1. The soothing movement of massage may ease tension and invoke a state of relaxation. There is some limited evidence that endorphins are released during massage which is said to help modify the pain experience and induce relaxation (Kaada and Torsteinbo 1989). Regular sessions may be required if there are long-standing physical and emotional problems to overcome.
2. The muscular system may be improved. Muscular wastage resulting from injury or paralysis cannot necessarily be prevented but may be ameliorated because muscle tone can be improved and muscular atrophy, resulting from enforced inactivity, can often be reduced. Massage is very useful for releasing chronic neck and shoulder tension. As long ago as the 1940s, Scull (1945) found that after massage there was a reduction of both muscle tension and muscle spasm. The increased blood supply encouraged by massage may help to reduce this spasm by eliminating waste products, such as uric acid, which accumulate in muscles and so relieve soreness, tension, stiffness and aches in both muscles and joints. Massage can also be used as a form of passive exercise that may partially compensate for lack of exercise, e.g. an arthritic patient may experience less pain by improving the peripheral circulation to their joints, especially when the inflammation is also moderated. Minor conditions such as bursitis and sprains respond readily to massage. Although it may be that back pain can be relieved, caution must be exerted when treating such pain (see below under 'Contraindications to massage').
3. The digestive system often benefits from massage. It is often useful for the minor discomforts associated with digestion, assimilation and elimination and I have found it to be helpful for those who are constipated. Beard and Wood (1994) found that abdominal massage increased peristaltic action.
4. The lymphatic system is improved by the application of deep effleurage. During massage its mechanical action aids tissue metabolism and the flow of lymph to the lymph glands is increased (Scull 1945). As a consequence of this, waste and toxins are more readily

flushed from the body. Sluggish lymph nodes may also be drained more efficiently. Mortimer (1990) found that localised and systemic lymphatic circulations are both improved by massage. Such treatment is very effective for reducing excess fluid in the legs and arms and for relieving swelling. This alone often relieves tired or aching limbs and helps rejuvenate tired and sore feet.

5. The respiratory system often benefits from a massage treatment because it has the potential to encourage respiratory muscles to relax, which may in turn aid deeper breathing. The symptoms associated with catarrh, nasal congestion and sinus conditions often respond dramatically and sometimes even disappear.

6. The nervous system benefits probably more from massage than any other system in the body, because it may be either soothed or stimulated, e.g. the gentle stroking of slow effleurage is calming and tension relieving to a nervous patient, whereas brisk effleurage may stimulate a sluggish system. Fraser and Ross Kerr's (1993) work noted that massage had the potential to reduce anxiety levels. Longworth (1982) noted how massage also helps patients cope with and in some cases overcome long-standing emotional turmoil and stress. Although many may see massage as a non-essential luxury, Hildebrand (1994) noted that:

> Emotionally massage can create a therapeutic 'space', relieving stress and allowing catharsis to occur.
>
> Hildebrand (1994)

It would therefore seem that it might be very valuable to consider as one of the treatment options for dealing with patients with emotional problems.

7. The circulatory system is said to benefit from massage. Longworth's (1982) study, conducted on 32 healthy women, demonstrated a significant reduction in anxiety, blood pressure and pulse rate after a slow back massage. The direct pressure of massage acts to stimulate the nerves that control the blood vessels and possibly because of this, when the local blood circulation is stimulated, it also generates some warmth (Kaada and Torsteinbo 1989).

8. Touch (see Chapter 2) alone may benefit the patient and also time spent with the patient.

Massage techniques

These are often described differently in different books. As a result of this I have chosen to use Arnould-Taylor's (1990) nomenclature.

Effleurage

The term 'effleurage' is derived from the French for flowing. The procedure starts when both hands are placed on the patient's body. Then, using
both hands, smooth, firm stroking movements are applied in an upward
direction towards the heart. Lighter downward movements, away from
the heart, immediately follow these. While performing any massage movement, the practitioner's hands should be in contact with the recipient at all
times. The hands should also mould to and follow the contours of the
patient's body so that continuous and rhythmical movements are made
during each sequence. Once the hands have returned to their starting
position the movement will be repeated several times. Although effleurage
is normally performed in a slow and rhythmical way to encourage relaxation and euphoria, it can also be executed briskly to stimulate a 'sluggish'
system. This movement can be used on all parts of the body and precedes
and succeeds all others to increase lymph and blood flow around the
massaged tissues (Figure 3.1 shows the direction of effleurage on the back).

Petrissage (some refer to this as friction)

This consists of small circular movements produced by rotating the balls
of the thumbs and/or fingers on the patient's body. Pressure is applied
directly to soft tissues and this pressure appears especially useful where
there is bone immediately underneath. Although this action needs to be

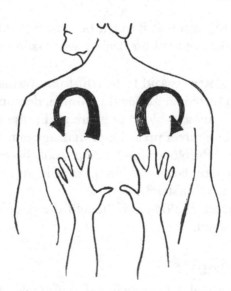

Figure 3.1 Direction of effleurage on the back.

quite firm and continuous, the amount of pressure required will depend on the patient's toleration of it or the part of the body involved, e.g. the amount of pressure exerted around the scapula is likely to be more than that applied to arthritic knuckles. It is both simple and effective, and its prime purpose is to 'break down' nodules, often referred to as adhesions or knotted muscle fibres, and aid toxin (waste product) elimination from soft tissues. It also helps increase the flow of blood to an area. Never use the fingertips for this movement and take care when performing this steady 'grinding' action so that the skin is trapped securely and friction is not induced. Petrissage can be quite painful to the thumbs of even experienced practitioners (Figure 3.2).

Kneading (some refer to this as petrissage)

Kneading (Figure 3.3) tends to be used on larger areas of the body, such as the inner thigh, where there is a high proportion of soft tissue and muscle and no bone immediately underneath. As its name indicates, it is similar to those actions used when kneading bread. The tissue is picked up with the fingers away from any bone and rolled back, using firm squeezing and wringing movements. The thumbs merely act as a gauge to the amount of pressure exerted. This again is dependent on the size of the muscle and the condition of the patient being treated, and should be performed only on warm and relaxed muscles. Kneading is especially effective in eliminating toxins or waste products from deep muscular tissue. It assists muscle contractability and the interchange of intracellular fluids, and is also said to break down fat (Arnould-Taylor 1990). In addition it is used in lymphatic drainage.

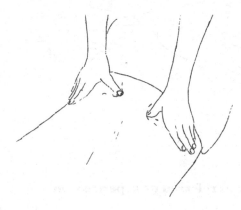

Figure 3.2 Petrissage.

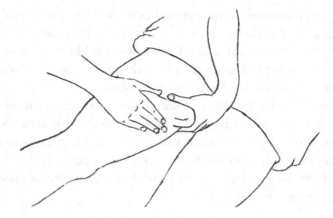

Figure 3.3 Kneading and wringing.

Hacking

This movement is likened to the action of the karate chop. Both hands are placed palms together as if you are about to pray. The hands should be relaxed and fingers loose. The outer edges of both hands then alternately and rhythmically move up and down and come into contact with the area of the body to be treated. It is used primarily to stimulate and tone large muscle groups, such as the upper thigh and back, shoulders and neck and should not be used where there is underlying superficial bone (Figure 3.4).

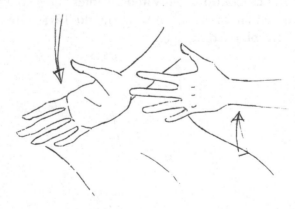

Figure 3.4 Hacking.

Cupping (sometimes referred to as percussion)

You will have seen this technique performed by physiotherapists. Both hands are cupped and applied rhythmically to the thighs, back and, in some cases, the buttocks. The movements start slowly and then increase in pace. If performed correctly the noise produced should sound hollow and has been likened to a horse trotting. This movement aims to produce a hyperaemic vacuum in order to increase superficial blood flow, stimulate peripheral nerve endings and aid the elimination of waste products from the muscles (Figure 3.5).

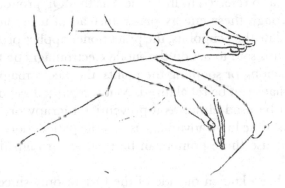

Figure 3.5 Cupping.

Tapotement

Tapotement tends to be used in beauty therapy rather more often than in massage therapy. It involves a flicking or tapping action of the pads of your fingers on small muscles such as those of the face, and requires very little practice to perfect. As well as being very relaxing for the recipient, it aids muscle tone.

In addition to being proficient in the above techniques it is also necessary to understand the significance of the amount of pressure to exert, the direction, rate and rhythm of the movements, and also the duration and frequency of treatment, before one can massage a patient expertly (Price and Price 1995).

Shiatsu

Shiatsu is worthy of a mention here. This is a traditional form of Japanese massage that aims to treat body, mind and spirit, and is said to be similar to Tui Na (Chinese acupressure). Its aim is therefore to trigger the body's self-regulating and healing systems. Both methods were developed from Amna, an ancient oriental system of rubbing and manipulation of both hands and feet. Shiatsu developed as a home treatment and although its knowledge was passed from one generation to another it did not become a formalised therapy until the early twentieth century. Tokujiro Namikoshi is said to be one of the first people to have popularised it.

Although Shiatsu means finger pressure, this therapy uses much more than that, because the practitioner also uses the heel and palms of his or her hands, elbows, knees and feet to exert pressure. This pressure is applied to the many 'tsubo' or surface points along the meridians, often referred to as energy paths. The aim of this treatment is to stimulate the flow of the 'Ki' (also referred to in Chinese as the 'Qi' pronounced 'chi') or life force through these energy paths. Instead of using acupuncture needles to stimulate the acupoints, the practitioner applies pressure to the specific points. It is said to act on the subtle electromagnetic fields of the body and, by exciting or soothing the points, the electromagnetic points along the meridians can be rebalanced. As it is regarded as both safe and effective, it can be used either as a preventive therapy or for treating specific ailments. One huge advantage is that the patient does not require undressing, because these points can be treated through the clothing (Davis 1999).

Shiatsu has been known outside of the Orient only since the 1970s and, although there are several types of Shiatsu practised, all are still based on the principles of traditional Chinese medicine. Training to become a Shiatsu practitioner takes upwards of 3 years, part time, and only those qualified in it should practise on patients (for a comprehensive introduction to Shiatsu, see Jarmey and Tschudin 1994).

Massage treatment

IF YOU HAVE ANY DOUBTS DO NOT MASSAGE

Before any treatment a case history must be taken in order that you may not only identify current problems requiring attention, but also past and current orthodox management. This then acts as a record of a patient's present and ongoing care and I have found the simple assessment sheet in Table 3.1 very useful.

Other preparation

Positioning

Having identified the patient's problem, explained the procedure and obtained informed consent, the patient should be positioned so that he or she is as comfortable as possible. You will need to adapt the procedure to suit the individual needs of your patient, e.g. those with breathing difficul-

Table 3.1 Assessment sheet

Name
Date of birth
Address
Tel:
GP   Tel:
Age:
Sex:
Occupation:
Height:
Lifestyle:
Weight:
Smoke:
Alcohol:

Medical history (including family history, previous illness, accidents, operations)
Current treatment and medication
Present illness/reason for consultation

Systems examination
Neurological
Cardiovascular
Respiratory
Digestive
Genitourinary/reproductive
Muscular
Skin
Signature of client (or another):
Initial treatment:[a]
Post-treatment: reactions, advice and date of next appointment

---

[a]Subsequent visits are then recorded on a separate continuation sheet.

ties may not be able to lie down for any length of time and those with arthritis and other painful conditions may need their position changed frequently. Patients who are very unwell and have debilitating chronic conditions such as chronic fatigue syndrome (often referred to as myalgic encephalopathy or ME) and HIV/AIDS may tolerate only very short sessions. Sometimes it is kinder to massage, perhaps, their arms or hands rather than attempt a whole body massage.

The massage sequence

This must be conducted in private and be undisturbed so that the patient will feel safe and secure throughout the whole procedure. While working with the patient you should aim to develop a good and trusting relationship. The room should be warm and quiet, and the massage is best performed on a comfortable firm surface, ideally a couch, to allow you to be able to maintain firm, regular, rhythmic movements. For continuity, once started, one of your hands should be in contact with the patient at all times. Only appropriate massage oil should be used (see below). Afterwards some time should be given to the patient to allow him or her to rest in this quiet and warm environment.

Pressure

This should be adjusted to accommodate the individual needs of your patient and it should be a pleasant rather than a painful experience. Do remember that the older the skin, the more friable it is likely to be, and that too vigorous and heavy a massage may cause further damage to an already fragile skin. This is especially so where it is also oedematous or dehydrated. There is also decreased strength and tone and some slowing of the response rate of muscles. In active elderly people, although there is some muscle atrophy the muscles will still be reasonably strong, but in inactive individuals the muscle fibres are even further reduced in both size and number. This may lead to fatty infiltration and even greater weakness which may be the result of motor neuron death, injury to muscle fibres, and also fewer and smaller mitochondria.

Massage oil

Only use a suitable massage oil and have this ready in a small bowl (Chinese dipping sauce containers are ideal for this because they are both attractive and relatively inexpensive), before commencing the procedure. Dip your fingers into the oil and warm the oil, by rubbing your hands together, before applying to the patient's body. Never drizzle oil directly on to the patient. The same procedure can also be adopted when using an essential oil blend (see Chapter 4).

Suitable massage oils

Any light seed, vegetable or nut oil may be used. Buy as good a quality oil as you can afford, but if you are unlikely to massage often buy only in small quantities because oils become rancid very quickly. These may also act as a carrier oil for essential oils (more is said about this in Chapter 4). Most therapists tend to use oil as a lubricant nowadays, but you may still see a therapist using talcum powder instead.

I prefer to use a relatively inexpensive, non-nut-based oil such as grape seed oil because of the current concerns about nut allergies. Although it seems that most allergic reactions to nuts reported in the press concern peanuts and are considered rare, Reading (1997), Director of the Anaphylaxis Campaign, disputes this. He feels that generally the public is ignorant of their potential danger. Yet, in ward settings, the peanut-derived arachis oil appears to be the most common one used by nurses in everyday practice. A research study reported in *The Lancet* (Pumphrey et al. 1998) found that individuals who are allergic to peanuts are also likely to react to other nuts. It is therefore imperative to be aware not only that some of our patients may be susceptible to nut allergies, but also that the younger nurses using it (or any babies they might have in the future) could also potentially be at risk. Other suitable oils for massage include avocado, calendula, evening primrose oil, jojoba (pronounced hohoba), safflower, sweet almond, sunflower and walnut (more is said about these in Chapter 4).

Post-treatment documentation

This should include details of the massage sequence, patient response and reactions and also any advice given.

The order of massage

As has already been said, the time spent on a massage will depend on the condition of the patient and how long he or she is able to tolerate it. Any massage is likely to include the various massage movements previously discussed (see above,) and it is essential to adopt a logical sequence so that the patient does not have to keep turning over.

I prefer to massage in the following order:

1. Lay the patient on his or her front (if able) and massage the lower then upper legs. Move up to the lower spine and then onto the upper back and neck.
2. Turn the patient over and massage the face (unless the patient chooses not to have this done), upper shoulders and front of arms down to include the fingers.
3. Massage the upper legs and then the lower legs, including the feet and toes.

Please note that I massage the abdomen only if the patient presents with constipation and I never massage the chest of either male or female patients. The exact order of massage is probably dependent on how the practitioner was taught.

Contraindications to massage

If appropriately practised massage is a safe procedure, but it is sometimes contraindicated. Although the list below details where total body massage is generally contraindicated, it may still be possible either to massage an unaffected part of the body or to use reduced pressure. Advice is given where this is possible.

Bruising

Treatments and conditions that cause easy bruising such as anticoagulant therapy, leukaemia, purpura and thrombocytopenia need to be assessed carefully. Very gentle massage may be possible.

Cardiovascular conditions

Where there is known cardiovascular disease, a history of thrombosis or phlebitis, whole body massage may be inadvisable because it may cause over-stimulation of an already weakened system, or if too vigorous it may move emboli. Although it is acceptable to massage around varicose veins, massage directly over them should be avoided, because normal pressure may cause damage to the blood vessels.

Confused patients

Such patients often respond well to touch but great care must be taken so that they are not startled or frightened by the massage and/or its after-effects.

Eating/Drinking

It is best not to massage immediately after the patient has consumed alcohol or a heavy meal.

Infection/Inflammation

Avoid massaging directly over any eruptions or contagious disease of the skin because massage may irritate or spread the condition. If the patient is suffering from an acute infection or inflammatory conditions, such as acute arthritis, neuritis, gastroenteritis or sunburn, he or she may not benefit from over-stimulation at this time.

Oncology

Although there are many myths surrounding the care of cancer patients, and massage is not necessarily contraindicated in those receiving oncology treatments, Hildebrand (1994) advises that it is likely that their skin will be hypersensitive to touch and consequently easily irritated. Therapists therefore need to be extra cautious and should always consult with physicians and radiotherapists responsible for the care of these patients before agreeing to massage. She advocates that whole body massage is inadvisable at this time because it may be too much for them to cope with. Extra caution is required for those who are undergoing chemotherapy or hormone therapy, because their skin may be very dry. Never massage directly over any cancerous lesion or the associated lymph nodes or massage until at least 10 days after radiation treatment. A specialist type of massage may be used to treat patients with lymphoedema. This usually combines manual lymphatic drainage with compression bandaging and should be offered only by those qualified to do so (Huit 2000).

Steroid therapy

Patients on steroid therapy should not receive a massage.

Temperature

Patients who are hypothermic should not be massaged because massage may increase peripheral circulation and reduce their core temperature even further. Those who are pyrexial may feel too unwell to benefit.

Unexplained pathology

All swellings, protuberances and inflammatory and painful conditions, including back pain, must be investigated and diagnosed before proceeding to massage.

Wounds

Recent wounds or sites of operations are generally best avoided especially where there is the danger of stretching scar tissue.

Hand and foot massage

Hand and foot massage can also be used effectively in situations either where a whole body massage may be too much for your frail and poorly patients to endure, or when time constraints would not allow it. Nurses need to be competent in these skills before they are performed on selected patients and must also abide by the conventions of normal massage practice (see above). Directly massaging the hands and/or feet may help to relieve and sometimes eliminate neuralgia and arthritic and rheumatic type pain.

When total body massage is contraindicated, the following hand and foot massage procedures may provide useful and realistic substitutes.

Hand massage

I have performed hand massage often and have also helped nurses to integrate it into their nursing care (Brett 1999). It can be performed using just a carrier oil or with the addition of suitably chosen essential oils (see Chapter 4). Hand massage is a very useful type of massage because hands are easily accessible and to experience it patients are not required to undress. It may also be more readily accepted than other types of massage because in this country it is commonplace to shake another's hand.

Although there is considerable anecdotal evidence about the advantages of hand massage, there is very little available research-based evidence. Price and Price (1995) noted how massage was both comforting and soothing, and Pietroni (1993) felt that it was both beneficial and harmless to practise as long as practitioners abided by the normal contraindications. Two small research studies, both conducted by the same American authors (Snyder et al. 1995a, 1995b), looked at the efficacy of hand massage and were supportive of its use in their aggressive, agitated client group and. although their findings were limited, they did show that these clients had benefited somewhat. In the first study the clients appeared more relaxed and in the second their aggressive behaviour was ameliorated

Suggested order of massage

1. Assess the patient and seek and obtain informed consent.
2. Wash your hands.
3. Position the patient and place a towel under his or her hands. Then smooth the oil on to the palms of your own hands and rub them together to warm it. Take the patient's first hand and sandwich it between your own two hands. Before attempting any massage movements allow the patient time to get used to your touch. When working on the hand always support it, either by allowing it to rest on the towel or by cradling it in one of your hands while massaging with the other.

4. Now use gentle effleurage type strokes covering the whole of both sides of the hand and remember to include the wrist and the thumb. Work up from the tips of the fingers towards the wrist (Figure 3.6). Repeat this movement several times.

5. Start to use petrissage on the patient's hand. Use both of your hands to perform these little thumb circles working mainly on the back of the hand. Do also work gently between the fronds of the fingers and thumb and pay special attention to the knuckles and thumb joint. Again work up from the tips of the fingers to the wrist. Repeat these movements several times

6. Turn the patient's hand over and gently petrissage all over the patient's palm several times. Afterwards rub gently along the solar plexus (in the middle of the palm), working from the centre of the wrist down the palm to the middle finger. This can be very soothing to the nervous system. Use alternate thumbs and repeat several times.

7. Depending on the patient, it may be useful, at this stage, to perform some passive exercise-type movements. First gently stretch each finger (Figure 3.7) then thumb, in turn, holding them gently between your finger and thumb and let your fingers slide from their knuckle down to their fingertips. Rotate each finger and the thumb twice in each direction. Then clasp and rotate the wrist clockwise and anti-clockwise. You have applied too much oil if your fingers slip during these actions! Repeat several times.

8. Finish by applying gentle effleurage to the whole hand.

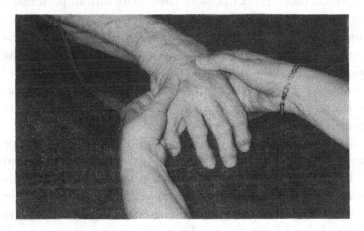

Figure 3.6 Effleurage of both sides of the hands

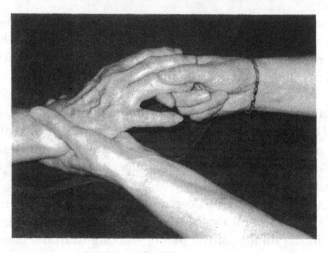

Figure 3.7 Stretching of fingers on an arthritic hand.

9. Repeat all movements on the patient's other hand.
10. Once both hands have been massaged, hold them both between your hands so that the treatment does not end abruptly.
11. Wash your hands and document all relevant information in the appropriate record.

Foot massage

Although I have less experience of this than hand massage, several studies appear to support its worth. Cox and Hayes (2000) investigated different ways in which they could massage their critically ill patients. As they could easily access such patients' feet and would not have to reposition them, unnecessarily, they chose foot massage with which to treat them. Their results showed that this 5-minute intervention was effective in the promotion of relaxation and in the amelioration of the effects of stress. The patients also revealed to them how much they looked forward to it, because it was so much nicer than any of the other interventions they had to endure!

Malkin (1994) documented the use of foot massage, alongside pethidine, with a patient who was suffering from post-surgical pain. She recorded that the patient's spinal pain was well controlled by the drug, but because of her anxiety she continued to experience muscle spasm around the site of the excision. While she admitted that her small case study was rather subjective, she did note that:

After 15 minutes of foot massage the patient was visibly relaxed and the muscle spasm and anxiety had decreased. The patient later stated that massage was the only thing which took the pain away.

Malkin (1994)

Order of massage

1. Assess the patient and seek and obtain informed consent.
2. Wash your hands.
3. Position the patient comfortably and place a towel under and over both feet. Make sure that they are clean and do not work on them if fungal infections are present. Uncover one foot and pour a little of your chosen oil into the palm of one hand. Rub your hands together to distribute and warm the oil evenly. Sandwich the foot between both hands (one on top and one underneath), then gently slide your hands over the foot and hold it for a while so that the patient gets used to your touch (Figure 3.8). The pressure you use needs to be firm enough so that it does not tickle but not so that it hurts. This, of course, will be dependent on your individual patient. Support the foot at all times during this procedure.

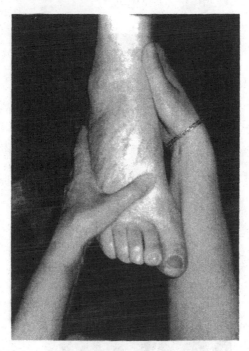

Figure 3.8 Holding the foot.

4. Commence slow and rhythmical effleurage and stroke firmly on the top of the foot from the toes to the ankle, then pass your hand around the ankle and, using a much lighter pressure, continue with this on the underside of the foot back to the toes. Repeat several times.

5. Then hold the inner and outer edges of the patient's foot with both hands and manipulate it from side to side (Figures 3.9 and 3.10). Use both of your thumbs to petrissage around the ankle, using gentle circular movements. As this area can be tender, work carefully and steadily. Repeat several times.

6. Carry on with the petrissage all over the top and sole of the foot with your thumbs, moving down from the ankle area to the toes. Repeat several times.

7. Depending on the patient, it may be useful, at this stage, to perform similar passive exercise-type movements to those used in the hand massage sequence. First gently stretch each toe, in turn, holding them gently between your finger and thumb and let your fingers slide from the ankle down to the tips of the toes. Rotate each toe twice in each direction. Then clasp and rotate the ankle clockwise and anti-clockwise. To finish off 'zig zag' down the sole of the foot from toes to heel

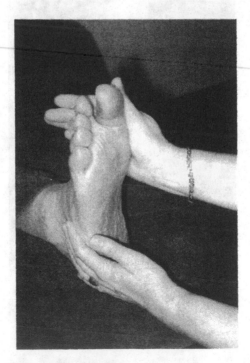

Figure 3.9 Holding the inner edge of the foot.

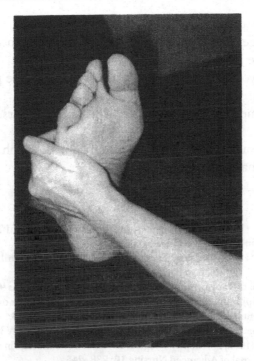

Figure 3.10 Holding the outer edge of the foot.

with your thumbs overlapped. Again you will have applied too much oil if your fingers slip during these actions! Repeat several times.

8. End by applying gentle effleurage to the whole foot.
9. Once completed, wrap the foot up again for warmth and repeat the movements on the other foot.
10. Once both feet have been massaged, hold them both between your hands so that the treatment does not end abruptly.
11. Wash your hands and document all relevant information in the appropriate record.

Massage is a very useful and effective therapy to use with older people. The exact order or choice of massage movements is not crucial as long as you take into account the individual condition and circumstances of your patients. Once you have gained some experience in this, the way you massage will become almost instinctual.

Questions

• Describe the massage movements and state when they would be used and why.

- What are the advantages of massage and why?
- Identify the general contraindications to massage and when a whole body massage is particularly contraindicated.
- How would you prepare the environment so that the patient will feel safe and secure during the massage treatment?
- Why do you need to take more care with an older person's skin during massage?
- Why might you choose a non-nut-based oil with which to lubricate the skin during massage?

References

Arnould-Taylor W (1990) The Principles and Practice of Physical Therapy, 2nd edn. Cheltenham: Stanley Thornes (Publishers) Ltd.

Beard G, Wood G (1994) Massage Principles and Techniques. Philadelphia, PA: WB Saunders.

Brett H (1999) Aromatherapy in the care of older people. Nursing Times 95(33): 56–57.

Cox C, Hayes J (2000) Immediate effects of a five minute foot massage on patients in critical care. Complementary Therapies in Nursing and Midwifery 6: 9–13.

Davis P (1999) Aromatherapy an A–Z, revised edn. Saffron Walden: CW Daniel Co. Ltd.

Fraser J, Ross Kerr J (1993) Psychophysiological effects of back massage in elderly institutionalized patients. Journal of Advanced Nursing 18: 238–245.

Goldstone L (2000) Massage as an orthodox medical treatment past and future. Complementary Therapies in Nursing and Midwifery 6: 169–175.

Hildebrand S (1994) Therapeutic massage and aromatherapy. In: Wells R, Tschudin V, eds, Wells' Supportive Therapies in Health Care. London: Baillière Tindall.

Hobbs S, Davies D (1998) Critical review of how nurses research massage therapy: are they using the best methods? Complementary Therapies in Nursing and Midwifery 4: 35–40.

Huit M (2000) Best practice. A guide to treating lymphoedema. Nursing Times 96(38): 42–43.

Jarmey C, Tschudin V (1994) Shiatsu. In Wells R, Tschudin V, eds, Wells' Supportive Therapies in Health Care, Chapter 7. London: Baillière Tindall, pp 130–152.

Kaada B, Torsteinbo O (1989) Increase of plasma beta endorphin levels in connective tissue massage. General Pharmacology 20: 487–489.

Longworth J (1982) Psychophysiological effects of slow stroke massage in normotensive females. Advances in Nursing Science 44–46.

Malkin K (1994) Clinical practice. Use of massage in clinical practice. British Journal of Nursing 3: 292–294.

Mortimer P (1990) The measurement of skin lymph flow by isotope clearance – reliability, reproducibility, injection dynamics and the effect of massage. Journal of Investigative Dermatology 95: 677–681 .

Pietroni J (1993) Massage. Nursing Times Special Issue Autumn: 62–69.

Price S, Price L (1995) Aromatherapy for Health Professionals. Edinburgh: Churchill Livingstone.

Pumphrey R, Wilson PB, Bansal AS (1998) Peanut allergy. The Lancet 352: 741–742.

Reading D (1997) Perspectives. Ticking time bomb. Nursing Standard 12(9): 16.

Scull C (1945) Massage – physiologic basis. Archives of Physical Medicine 26: 159–167.

Snyder M, Egan E, Burns K (1995a) Efficacy of hand massage in decreasing agitation behaviors associated with rare activities in people with dementia. Geriatric Nursing March/April: 60–63.

Snyder M, Egan E, Burns K (1995b) Interventions for decreasing agitation behaviors in persons with dementia. Journal of Gerontological Nursing July: 35–40.

Vickers A (1996) Massage and Aromatherapy: A guide for health professionals. London: Chapman & Hall.

CHAPTER 4
Aromatherapy

Look in the perfumes of flowers and of nature for peace of mind and joy of life.

Wang-Wei (eighth-century AD)

Aromatherapy is the use of aromatic substances (mainly essential oils) that have been extracted from plants, in a controlled way, for therapeutic effect and it has become, possibly, one of the fastest growing therapies within both the UK and many other parts of the world (Tisserand and Balacs 1995). The aim is to achieve physical, mental and spiritual equilibrium by the harmonising and balancing effects of these oils. Therefore some have claimed that it is not only a holistic therapy that encompasses health promotion and disease prevention, but also a safe and natural alternative to drugs (Brown 1993)!

The term 'aromatherapie' (aromatherapy) was first coined by the French chemist René-Maurice Gattefosse in 1928 while researching the use of oils for the cosmetic trade. During one of his laboratory experiments, there was a small explosion and he burnt his hand. He immediately plunged the injured hand into a vat of lavender oil and was surprised to discover that it healed quickly without leaving a scar. Following this discovery Gattefosse carried out further research on soldiers in World War II. He found that the wounds he treated with essential oils healed very quickly even though the soldiers continued to stay at the battlefront. Although Jean Valnet was influential in developing the use of essential oils, it was the Austrian Marguerite Maury who first blended these oils so that they could be used initially in beauty therapy. Since the 1960s they have been used in the UK for therapeutic purposes as well.

The origins of aromatherapy

The use of plant extracts for healing began centuries ago in the ancient Greek, Roman, Indian, Chinese, Egyptian, Australian aboriginal and Persian civilisations, and is also referred to in the Bible. The Egyptians most famously used them in a variety of ways. Records dating back to 4500 BC reveal how aromatic plants were used for cosmetics, as perfumes, medicinally and for embalming the dead in preparation for the after-life. Hopkins (1995) notes how traces of clove, nutmeg, cinnamon and cedarwood were found in the bandages of the mummified Pharaohs, and other oils were present in the tomb of the young King Tutankhamun (1361–1352 BC), when it was opened in 1922. Further evidence of their use is the burning of oils shown in the early Egyptian hieroglyphics.

Oils such as cinnamon, cassia and myrrh are mentioned within the writings of both Testaments of the Bible. The most famous of these is in St Matthew's Gospel in the New Testament, where the story of the Three Wise Men bringing the precious frankincense and myrrh to the newly born baby Jesus is recounted (Stevensen 1995):

> And when they were come into the house, they saw the young child with Mary his mother, and fell down and worshipped him: and when they had opened their treasures, they presented unto him gifts; gold, and frankincense, and myrrh.
>
> Chapter 2, verse 11

Throughout the ages other cultures also became involved with their use and this oft-quoted phrase by the great physician Hippocrates (460–370 BC) seems to encapsulate the philosophy behind the practice of aromatherapy:

> The way to health is to have an aromatic bath and scented massage every day.
>
> Cited in Maxwell-Hudson (1988)

But it was in Arabia, during the eleventh century, that the Persian physician Avicenna re-introduced the process of distilling essential oils, which continues to be used today (Hopkins 1995). During the Crusades trade routes were increasingly opened up and the knights brought back with them essential oils to Europe. At this time these perfumed oils were used to mask smells and also to ward off infection. It is thought that the nursery rhyme 'Ring a ring a roses' (in the line 'A pocket full of posies') is referring to their use. Other customs, such as the wearing of orange blossom (neroli) in the hair of brides on their wedding day, is said to originate from this time. Between the thirteenth and seventeenth centuries most of the essential oils as we know them today had been discovered. But in the eighteenth and nineteenth centuries the production of synthetic, and somewhat toxic, oils for pharmaceutical as opposed to medicinal use began. This, coupled with the rise of drug synthesis, led to a decline in the popularity of essential oils.

Essential oils

Although aromatic plants and their extracts have been used for many thousands of years in medicines and cosmetics, distilled essential oils are much newer and deemed to be more potent. Their chemical make-up and quality are dependent on how and where they are cultivated and also on their manufacture. Each oil is made up of the following key components: terpenes (hydrocarbons); oxygenated compounds such as esters, aldehydes, alcohols, phenols, oxides, aldehydes and ketones; and in some instances sulphur, nitrogen and lactones. Tisserand and Balacs (1995, page 8) wrote that:

> . . . a typical essential oil is a complex mixture of over 100 different chemical compounds, created and mixed by the parent plant. These have related but distinct types of chemical structure and give the oil its smell, its therapeutic properties in and, some cases, its toxicity. Many of them are extremely widespread throughout the plant kingdom, and many essential oils share some of the same ingredients. Some essential oil constituents are present in only trace amounts; if sufficiently potent they may still be important ingredients, either therapeutically or toxicologically.
>
> Tisserand and Balacs (1995)

Although their precise action on the body is unknown it is crucial to recognise their uniqueness and identify them accurately. Franchomme and Penoel (1990) advocate that the correct Latin botanical name should always be given because the therapeutic properties of a subspecies of plant may differ from the original genus. They use lavender as an example of this and stress that, whereas the chemical composition of *Lavandula angustifolia* (true lavender) has no known side effects and is deemed safe to use, *Lavandula stoechas*, because of its potentially toxic composition, may not be. Although Tisserand and Balacs (1995) assert that, used properly, most essential oils signify little or no risk to an individual, they do state that, because there is such complex information surrounding them, some of the advice given, inevitably 'involves subjective judgment' (page 3).

Davis (1999) reminds us that it is an essence that is produced from the plant and that this becomes an essential oil only after it has been processed by distillation, and yet this term is often used inaccurately to describe all the volatile oils used in aromatherapy. Therefore, technically speaking, those oils that are produced by expression, such as citrus oils, are really still an essence and others such as jasmine and rose obtained by enfleurage and solvent extraction, should be termed 'absolutes'.

As a result of the name aromatherapy, it is often thought that benefit comes only from inhalation of these odiferous smells. The essential oils are, however, able to enter the body by two other routes as well, namely via the skin and by internal application.

Internal use

Essential oils used internally may irritate the gastric mucosa and are said to be more likely to cause systemic damage because they reach the bloodstream more readily than those administered externally (Tisserand and Balacs 1995). Although the French commonly ingest oils in various forms (Valnet 1990) and several books and articles do advocate this, because of the concerns within UK aromatherapy organisations about their potential danger, they currently do not allow their members to use essential oils internally. The Aromatherapy Organisations Council (AOC) in 1998 gave the following unpublished directive:

> The AOC does not permit treatment via oral ingestion of essential oils by qualified aromatherapy practitioners of its member associations unless they are also suitably qualified to the equivalent standard of a medical herbalist or a medical doctor.
>
> AOC (1998)

A qualified non-doctor member of one of these organisations would be able to obtain insurance only for oils used externally. As the use of essential oils for oral ingestion does not come within the range of professional nursing practice, it is not addressed in this book.

Inhalation

Two things occur when essential oils are inhaled. One is the inhalation of odorous molecules into the respiratory tract and the other is the recognition of their unique smells during the olfactory process.

Inhalation into the respiratory tract

Broadly speaking, after inhalation of these vapours into the nose, they will travel down into the lungs, via the bronchi and bronchioles to the alveoli, where gaseous exchange will take place. Inevitably some of these molecules will be lost into the general circulation, but as the surface of the lung is so large many will be absorbed by it and enter the bloodstream. The amount of uptake of these vapours is entirely dependent on the rate and depth of breathing. This route is seen as an effective treatment route because absorption of the gaseous molecules is almost instantaneous and very few ill-effects have been noted. As a result of this, even when patients are anosmic, they are thought to be able to benefit from the therapeutic properties of essential oils (Price and Price 1995).

Olfaction and smell

The sense of smell is less well understood than the other senses and, although its role is not as significant in humans as it is in animals, it is necessary to understand the mechanism and evocative nature of smell before contemplating the use of essential oils. The organ of smell is the olfactory mucosa of the nose. This yellowish tissue covers the superior concha, the roof of the nasal cavity and the upper part of the nasal septum. Inhaled air passes below the olfactory mucosa and as you sniff air is brought into contact with the nasal receptor cells; it is this that helps you smell an odour.

The mucosa is quite complex and contains receptor cells that are actually bipolar neurons. Their dendrites form not only the olfactory rods, which end in fine cilia, but also the supporting cells, the microvilli of which secrete mucus. These supporting cells and the Bowman's glands produce a pigment, which appears to be integral to the appreciation of smell. The inhaled odorous airborne molecules of a scented substance combine with smell receptors on the surface of the cilia, and they must dissolve in the nasal mucus before they are able to stimulate these receptors. It is unknown how smells are differentiated, but it is likely that variations in the smell receptors, the olfactory mucosa or the length of time between each successive stimulus could be responsible.

Essential oils are very volatile and therefore, when exposed to air, they evaporate into vapour and, because the inside of the nose is always moist, when these vapours are breathed in they dissolve readily. The aromatic particles can be detected only by the olfactory nerves in this form. The brain is able to identify the individual smell only after the neural fibres have passed this information to it. This is an instantaneous process which enables us to perceive the smell as soon as we are in contact with it, although, if the 'docking depression' that receives each individual aroma is missing, the smell will not be registered (Price and Price 1995). There are various degrees of anosmia and most people will experience some loss of smell at some time. This loss may be permanent or transitory and in some instances odour specific. Although it is not clear whether aromatherapy is less beneficial to anosmic patients, Davis (1999) feels that, although they may not experience such a total emotional response, they will gain something from their therapy because of the inevitable absorption of these oils through their skin and lungs.

The sense of smell is transmitted by the olfactory (cranial I) nerve and its connections (although irritant smells such as ammonia are transmitted via the trigeminal (cranial V) nerve). As these olfactory nerves lie in the upper part of the nose and are directly connected to the brain, the sense of smell is not only the most instantaneous of our senses but also the most fleeting. Some writers also believe that the thresholds for smell increase with age (Riley and Foner 1968). Stimulation of these smell receptors triggers a reaction within the olfactory epithelium, which is made up of 20 000 000 nerve endings, where it is transmuted into a nerve message. This is then amplified by the olfactory bulb and the resultant nerve impulse is then transmitted along the nerve fibres, through the cribriform plate, to the olfactory bulb. This message is then amplified by the olfactory bulb and from here information about the smell is relayed to the limbic system in the temporal lobe of the cerebral cortex.

Although it is known that smells are carried via the olfactory system and are processed in the limbic system, it is unclear to what extent smells affect our emotions and memories or how exactly olfaction takes place. Davis (1999) asserts that, because smell is registered in the limbic area of the brain, it shows that there is a direct link between odour and the psyche. It must therefore also assume a primary function in those emotions that are associated with pain, pleasure, anger, rage, fear, sorrow, sexual feelings, docility and affection. Although this system is regarded as being responsible for processing our emotions and is sometimes referred to as the visceral or emotional brain, the link between smell and emotions remains tenuous.

It does seem, however, that memories and their associations with smells are consciously learnt and once learnt very hard to forget, e.g. when I was a first year student nurse, on my second ward, one particular baby frightened me probably because she made such awful noises and also because her care was so demanding. Even now, many years later, when I smell the soap with which I washed her, the memories come flooding back! On the other hand, different smells will, very often, trigger much happier memories.

The skin (see Chapter 3 for the age-related changes)

The skin is the body's largest organ and, because of this, it is one of the two major routes by which essential oils may enter the bloodstream (the other, the lung, has been discussed above). Skin is also a major excretory organ and is therefore able to get rid of waste products easily, through the sweat. As the molecular structure of most essential oils is quite simple and they are often very small, they are able to pass through the skin relatively easily and into the bloodstream to give a systemic effect. The fact that they are readily dissolved in the skin's sebum makes absorption easier. This action is thought to be similar to that of fat-soluble drugs. Topically applied chemical substances may not, however, be absorbed into the body via the skin as efficiently in older populations because of the changes in the microcirculation. In the main, essential oils are metabolised in the liver and excreted via the kidneys and bladder, although clove is said to be excreted via the lungs. In addition to the therapeutic properties that they may possess, many are also able to help to nourish the skin (see Appendix I for examples).

One small study by Jager et al. (1992) is suggestive of a link between inhalation and skin penetration. They studied the percutaneous absorption of the essential oil lavender (specific genus not isolated), in males, after a massage. The results showed that the oil had penetrated the skin and that traces of linalyl and linalyl acetate, two of the main constituents of lavender, were present in the blood within 5 min of completing the massage. After a further 85 min, the study also revealed that most of the oil had been eliminated. They concluded that the relaxation and sedation experienced, post-massage, was probably as a result of both inhalation and penetration through the skin.

Methods of extraction

During plant photosynthesis concentrated oils are produced. These oils are stored in specific cells or reservoirs in different parts of the plant (Worwood 1994) and can be gathered from diverse sources. They are extracted from leaves (rosemary), flowers (rose), fruit (lemon), root (ginger), gum (frankincense), wood (sandalwood), beans (tonka bean) and seeds (fennel). Various oils may be produced from one plant, e.g. the orange tree produces neroli from its blossom, petigrain from its leaves and orange from its zest.

Different methods are employed to obtain the essential oils and the most common ones are listed below.

Distillation (steam or water)

Most oils are produced in this way and those that are distilled are deemed to be the most pure. Huge vats are filled with the chosen plants and then pressurised steam or water is passed over them. This process causes a vaporisation of the oils. On cooling the oils condense and, as essential oils are not water soluble, they are easily separated and collected for use. The aromatic water that is left is not discarded but may be sold as a byproduct for the perfume industry. In some instances the distillation process is reduced and an inferior quality oil is produced, which may be potentially more irritating than a 'pure' oil (Stevensen 1995). Even the most stringently produced oils may, however, be contaminated because of global pollution and the likelihood of some pesticide residue breaching the distillation barrier.

Enfleurage

Enfleurage, not to be confused with the massage term 'effleurage', is often used for the more expensive and fragile flowers such as jasmine and rose. The heat and pressure of the distillation process would be too harsh for such flowers and would spoil the resulting essential oils. The flowers are layered between unadulterated cold fat and left until the fat absorbs their perfume. After repeating this process several times, the fat is purified by rinsing with alcohol and heating gently. The resultant oil is usually very expensive because of the labour-intensive method of its production. It is widely quoted, for instance, that it takes 30 rose heads to make one drop of oil and 8 million jasmine flowers to manufacture only 1 kilogram of the essential oil!

Expression

Expression (or pressing) as its name suggests involves the squeezing of oil from the rind of mostly citrus fruits. Manufacturers tend to use machines nowadays to extract these oils, because it is now no longer economically viable to produce sufficient quantities by hand.

Extraction

Solvent extraction is a highly complex procedure that involves the use of solvents such as petroleum or alcohol to extract the essential oils. It is mainly used for gums and resins that are initially covered with the solvent and heated. The oils obtained are then cooled and filtered. As it is difficult to ensure that the resultant oil is 'pure' and free from all solvents, they are referred to as absolutes. This method is used widely in the perfume industry.

Carrying media

Skin application

As essential oils are too concentrated to apply directly to the skin, they are first diluted in a carrying medium.

Carrier or base oils for massage

There is a vast assortment of non-volatile oils from which to choose. Some are suitable to use alone but others are better mixed together as a blend. Most oils may be used as a base and sometimes even unrefined cooking oils are used. The best ones are those that are labelled 100% extra virgin, pure refined or cold pressed, and should have little or no aroma. Oils not labelled in this way are normally extracted by heat or solvent processes and have had their trace elements and minerals destroyed. Baby oil is generally considered unsuitable because it is felt to impede the essential oils' absorption through the skin because of its low penetrability. Sweet almond and grapeseed oils are both reasonably priced and are widely used (see Chapter 3 for information relating to nut allergies).

Although there are many oils on general sale, those listed below are readily available and valuable to use:

- Avocado is a dark-green, nourishing and relatively expensive oil that contains fatty acids, protein, lecithin and vitamins, and is especially useful for patients with dry and dehydrated skin. As a result of its heaviness it is best used as an additive (in a 10% dilution) to one of the cheaper base oils.
- Calendula is a relatively expensive, macerated or infused oil that is better added to the main carrier oil (in a 10% dilution) than used alone. It is a rather thick and heavy oil but is useful for nourishing and healing the skin.
- Evening primrose oil is another relatively expensive oil. It is pale yellow and contains vitamins, minerals and gamma-linolenic acid. It is particularly useful for menopausal problems and is said to help patients with heart disease, multiple sclerosis and psoriasis. It is best added to another carrier oil (in a 10% dilution).

- Grapeseed is inexpensive, odourless, and often highly refined and pale green in colour. It is rich in vitamins and minerals and, as it is suitable for all skin types, is extensively used on its own.
- Jojoba (pronounced hohoba), which is actually a wax, is an expensive yellow 'oil' produced from beans. When cold it remains wax-like and contains protein, minerals, vitamin E and a substance that is said to mimic collagen. As a result of this it is particularly useful for sensitive skins and dermatological conditions but is best used as part of a blend (in a 10% dilution).
- Safflower is a useful general base oil because it is inexpensive and suitable for all skin types. It is pale yellow and contains vitamins, minerals and protein, and may be used alone.
- Sweet almond is an inexpensive, pleasing, pale yellow oil. It is often used on its own because it is very easily obtained, has an agreeable aroma and feels lovely on the skin. It is rich in protein and suitable even for sensitive and inflamed skin.
- Walnut oil is a sticky, relatively inexpensive oil and is especially useful for massage because it is high in unsaturated fatty acids.

Methods of use

Massage (for massage techniques and therapeutic benefits see Chapter 3)

This is a very effective way to use essential oils because it is believed that, after the essential oils penetrate the skin, they are absorbed into the bloodstream and travel to other systems. When applied to the skin the essential oils must be diluted in a carrier oil and used sparingly. Price and Price (1995) state, quite rightly, that, although those who practise aromatherapy are not necessarily trained or skilled in remedial massage, it should not deter them from applying oils to the skin. They assert that, by learning a few basic strokes and the contraindications for massage, the prime aim of enabling the absorption of the essential oil can be achieved. The ratio of essential oil to carrier oil is dependent on the age and condition of the patient. Generally, three to four different essential oils are sufficient to use on a client in one blend and if they are combined together a synergistic blend is produced. Worwood (1994) advocates that the dilution should be no more than 1 drop of essential oil per 1 millilitre of base oil, yet other therapists, including myself, prefer to use only 3–4 drops of essential oil to each 10 ml of base oil.

Other ways to use essential oils

Apart from including them in your massage, essential oils can be used in the bath, as an inhalant, in creams and also mouth salves and washes, as most of the oils are multipurpose. Probably the best example of this is lavender (*Lavandula angustifolia*) as it is so versatile and is used to treat pain, circulatory, digestive, muscular, respiratory, skin and neurological conditions. A few more specific examples include peppermint (*Mentha piperita*), black pepper (*Piper nigrum*) and rosemary (*Rosemarinus officinalis*) for physical symptoms such as pain; ginger (*Zingiber officinale*) for sickness; peppermint (*Mentha piperita*) for indigestion; marjoram (*Origanum marjorana*) for constipation and lemon (*Citrus limonum*) for fluid retention. Although in general respiratory disorders such as coughs, colds and sinusitis respond to cajuput (*Melaleuca leucadendron*), eucalyptus (*Eucalyptus globulus*) and tea tree (*Melaleuca alternifolia*), neurological and emotional events benefit from mood-enhancing oils such as jasmine (*Jasminum officinale*), rose (*Rosa damascena*) and ylang ylang (*Cananga odorata*).

Bathing

This is another effective way of using essential oils and it is particularly useful as an aid to relaxation or sleep and as a means of easing general aches and pains. The oils may be added directly to the bath water or dissolved in a carrier oil if the patient is very sensitive. Remember that adding essential oils directly to water does not dilute them. Davis (1999) suggests that instead of using a carrier oil to dilute them you could use full cream milk, before putting them in the bath. A while ago one of my post-registration students did advise me to try this. Whether added directly to the water or as part of a blend, the water needs to be agitated to disperse the mix evenly. Make sure also that no oil splashes in the eyes. To minimise evaporation of the oils, the bath water should be warm and run before the addition of the oils. It is safe to bathe with oils daily and the maximum effect is achieved by staying in the water for 15–20 min at a time. Not only will bathing in warm water aid direct absorption of the oils through the skin, but also indirectly via inhalation of the vapours. Between 5 and 6 drops, either as a single oil or combination of oils, are sufficient for an adult's bath.

Foot/sitz/hand bath

If patients are unable to get in or out of a full-size bath, treatments may be adapted to accommodate them in a localised bath. Although foot and hand baths are very useful for relieving sore and painful or inflammatory conditions, a sitz bath, for sitting in, as its name suggests, is especially helpful for easing rectal and vaginal conditions. Normally 4 drops of essential oil, singly or in combination, would be added to the water. Make sure the oil is well dispersed so that no globules come into contact with any delicate area.

Inhalation

The inhalation route is extremely useful, not only for relieving congestion, catarrh and most respiratory conditions, but also as another route for administering essential oils. There are very many simple ways in which patients may benefit from this and a few are listed below:

- Put 2 drops of neat oil, such as cajuput (*Melaleuca leucadendron*) or eucalyptus (*Eucalyptus globulus*), on a handkerchief or tissue to ease sinusitis, or cold and flu symptoms.
- Put 2 drops of neat lavender (*Lavandula angustifolia*) oil on a pillow to help an insomniac sleep.
- Two to three drops of essential oils may be added to a bowl of hot water and inhaled. The patient is encouraged to lean over the bowl, with a towel over his or her head, and breathe in the steaming vapours for a few moments. The patient should close the eyes and inhale deeply for up to 10 min or for as long as he or she is able. This is particularly useful for troublesome secretions and the treatment may be repeated several times a day. An ideal piece of apparatus to use would be the Nelson's inhaler, but unfortunately there are few of these about now! Great care must be taken when using this method, with vulnerable individuals, because it is potentially very dangerous. Such treatment may need to be closely supervised.
- Two drops of peppermint (*Mentha piperita*) and 2 drops of cajuput (*Melaleuca leucadendron*) may be added to 10 ml of grapeseed oil and used as a rub. It may be applied to the chest, or under the nose and throat to act as a decongestant.

Essential oils may also be administered via commercially available oil burners and vaporisers. These warm the essential oils and release their fragrant molecules into the atmosphere. The former are unlikely to be allowed within institutions because they rely on a naked candlelight to heat the oil in the bowl and the latter, before use, must comply with the institutions' safety policy regarding electrical appliances.

Compresses

These are very useful to ease strains, aches and pains and febrile conditions. To a small bowl of warm or cold water add 1–2 drops of essential oil. After mixing well immerse a muslin square, a cotton handkerchief or a flannel in the water, then wring out. Place the damp cloth on the affected part and leave for a few moments. Repeat as necessary.

Miscellaneous

Essential oils may be added to other carrying media and used in a variety of ways.

Mouth washes and lip salves

For insurance purposes, these are not considered internal applications. Several essential oils are useful for treating conditions of the mouth and these include myrrh (*Commiphora myrrha*) because of its anti-fungal properties and tea tree (*Melaleuca alternifolia*) for its anti-bacterial and immunostimulant properties

To make a mouth wash add 2 drops (in total) of essential oils per half tumbler of lukewarm water and make clear to patients that, once they have gargled with the mixture, they are not to swallow it.

One to two drops of essential oil, such as myrrh (*Commiphora myrrha*), added to 50 g of a good quality cream makes a useful salve that can be applied to sore and cracked lips.

Cream bases

Different base creams are available commercially in which to blend essential oils. Creams are useful when preparing a blend for patients for self-application, because they are less sticky and more manageable than base oils.

Lotions

Small amounts of essential oils may also be added to cleanser, liquid soap, bath, shower, shampoo and conditioner gels.

Floral waters

These may be made up and used either as a perfume or as a room freshener. The essential oils are added to a water spray bottle and sprayed as required. Care must be taken to avoid the eyes or polished surfaces.

Treatments

In all cases the essential oil will be chosen according to individual need after careful assessment of both the patient and his or her condition. Treatment should be provided using the most logical sequence and route of application and then appropriately documented (see Chapter 3 for sample assessment sheet).

Therapeutic effects

Although Mantle (1999) and Vickers (1996) both note that within the literature there is confusion and also lack of agreement about not only the therapeutic properties, but also the toxicity and administration of essential oils, Hopkins (1995) feels that this is not detrimental to care but just showed an individual therapist's preferred oil and mode of treatment. Valnet (1990) asserts that even this lack of firm evidence should not necessarily mar their value in healing. Although Stevensen (1995) recognises that there is currently a lack of rigorous published research into therapies such as aromatherapy and that their use should be rationalised, she feels that they should not be discounted, because they have been influential in traditional healthcare systems for more than 2000 years.

Contraindications/Precautions (contraindications when using specific essential oils are given in Appendix I)

1. DO NOT DABBLE (Mackereth 1995, Stevensen 1995). Although essential oils are freely available in supermarkets and health food shops they are all potentially hazardous to use. It is crucial therefore to be adequately trained in their application before they are used on patients. They all need to be administered cautiously because they are deemed to be between 70% and 90% more potent than the herbs, plants, trees, etc. from which they are derived. As each essential oil has its own specific therapeutic properties and actions, it needs to be chosen according to the particular needs of each patient because certain oils will be contraindicated for some but not for others (this will be considered in more depth in Part III when discussing treatment). If there is some doubt about which oil to use, it is better to err on the side of caution and select another. Tisserand and Balacs (1995) give very specific advice about essential oils contraindicated for both individual disease and also route of application (see also Appendix II for hazardous essential oils).

2. Do not use internally (see above).

3. Do not use neat essential oils. Although some oils can be used neat on the skin, it is not generally recommended and it is vital to check carefully before doing so as many will cause skin irritation. The two essential oils that seem to be used neat are lavender (*Lavandula angustifolia*) and tea tree (*Melaleuca alternifolia*), but they should be used like this only for first aid purposes. If using in this way, place just one drop on the affected area. Even those oils that are deemed safe to use on the skin should, however, first be tested. Place 1 drop of the chosen oil on the inner thigh and leave overnight. If there is any sensitivity to the oil, an allergic reaction, in the form of a rash or generalised redness, will appear.

4. Avoid the eyes and be extra careful with mucous membranes even when using diluted essential oils.

5. Avoid the over-use of the same oils to prevent yourself or your client from becoming accustomed and possibly resistant to their therapeutic benefits.

6. Take extra care with sensitive skin. Several oils, although useful for inhalation, may be irritating to the skin. The picture is not, however, totally clear on this because different practitioners have different views about what should not be used, e.g. although Tisserand and Balacs (1995) and Price and Price (1995) both document that clove bud (*Syzygium aromaticum*) is a dermal irritant, but safe to use in low concentrations, unless there is skin disease or hypersensitivity present, Davis (1999) feels that it should not be used at all on the skin. Most authors do tend to agree that all the citrus oils are potential dermal irritants and must be used with caution. If in doubt use another oil.

7. Avoid applying essential oils before using a sunbed or going out in the sun because they may cause increased photosensitivity to ultraviolet light and even cause burning of the skin. Davis (1999) states that dilutions of less than 2% do not appear to do this.

8. Store carefully and keep away from children and other vulnerable populations.

9. Use 'pure' essential oils in properly diluted solutions and do not overdose. The precise dilution will vary according to the specific essential oil chosen and the condition of the patient.

10. Remember that oils vaporised into the atmosphere will be inhaled by not only the selected recipient, but also others in the immediate vicinity!

11. Do not use on an open wound and take care over varicose veins.

12. Do not massage (contraindications to massage are presented in Chapter 3) when fever is present because it is thought that the patient may be over-stimulated.
13. Do not use aromas that people do not like because they may evoke a poor psychological response or trigger a forgotten unpleasant memory.

Buying and storage

Even the cheaper essential oils are relatively expensive and, even though their aroma may still be present, they lose their therapeutic properties very quickly. Although a couple of oils such as frankincense and sandalwood are said to mature and improve with age and unopened oils may last up to 6 years, once opened most oils are said to have only a limited shelf-life. Citrus oils are thought to retain their properties for only about 6 months because they become cloudy through oxidation and, depending on the genus, between 1 and 2 years for the others. Blended oils are effective for only up to 3 months.

As there is no definition of, or standard for, essential oil quality, it is extremely difficult to decide just how safe or pure any oil is. It is sensible, therefore, to buy oils in small quantities from reputable suppliers, replace them as and when you need to, and look after them properly. Prices do vary enormously depending on the type and quality of the oil available, e.g. my supplier's current catalogue lists *Eucalyptus globulus* at £1.90 for 50 ml, but half the quantity of *Melissa officinalis* for £450, exclusive of VAT!

As essential oils are highly volatile, affected by light and evaporate easily, they need careful storage. To help retain their properties, they should ideally be bottled in brown glass and kept, securely closed in their original containers, in a dry, cool, dark place. Plastic should not be used because it may have a detrimental effect on the essential oils. I prefer them, for safety reasons, to have dropper inserts, to be labelled clearly with both botanic and common names, and to state that they are not for ingestion. They need also to be kept out of the way of anyone who is vulnerable. Currently, there is no legal requirement to do any of this.

Issues associated with introducing essential oils into orthodox settings

It would be much easier, in my opinion, for health professionals to use essential oils in healthcare settings if manufacturers of essential oils followed health service dictates in the packaging of their products, e.g. when I tried to help nurses from two elderly continuing care wards to introduce aromatherapy into their daily practices, there were some initial safety and administrative problems to overcome (Brett 1999). The two main issues that had to be considered involved teaching the nurses to be competent to practise and ensuring the safety of the chosen essential oils. The first issue was relatively easy to address because I had been asked by the ward staff to help them develop an aromatherapy hand massage programme, and they were therefore keen both to learn and to practise the necessary skills. The senior nurses were first taught the procedure by me and then took on the responsibility for cascading them down to the more junior members of their nursing team.

The matter of essential oil safety was far more complex. I made up the essential oil and carrier blend, as the pharmacy was reluctant to be involved because not only were there no expiry dates on the bottles but also written safety information accompanying these oils was either generally unavailable or mostly inadequate. As a result of this, Fowler and Wall (1997, 1998) noted just how difficult it is to carry out the necessary Control of Substances Harmful to Health (COSHH 1994) and Chemical Hazard Information and Packaging for Supply (CHIPS 1996) assessments. Although they acknowledge that the risks of using essential oils may be 'less significant' than other chemicals, they assert that, as the practice of aromatherapy is mostly unregulated, it is vital that it meets the requirements of the Health and Safety at Work Act (HASAWA), so that it may protect both the users and the recipients of such potentially harmful substances (Fowler and Wall 1998). They also stressed that any risk assessment is the responsibility of the practitioner concerned! Bearing this in mind, I still continue to make up the oils for them and, although this project has not been formally evaluated, as yet the ward environment appears calmer for both the patients and nurses involved.

Aromatherapy is said to be a holistic therapy, but it can be this only if the whole needs of your individual patients are considered. This means that your assessment must consider their physical, psychological, emotional and spiritual needs, and this is never more challenging than when caring for dying patients and their grieving relatives (more is said about this later). Used skilfully, this therapy has the potential to help patients, relatives and carers to cope with chronic illness, the dying process and also to help the newly bereaved face the future more positively. If used wisely aromatherapy may bring not only joy to your patients but also comfort to you.

Questions

Try to answer the following questions:

1. What is an essential oil and how is it thought to work?
2. What is the difference between an essential oil and a carrier oil?
3. What do you need to consider when buying and storing both essential and carrier oils?
4. Look in Appendix I and try to identify the most appropriate essential oil to use for the following conditions: headache, insomnia, respiratory congestion and constipation. Why would you choose these oils and what would be the preferred route for their application?
5. Identify and describe the ways in which essential oils are manufactured.
6. Why did the use of aromatic plants for healing decline in the early part of the nineteenth century and who were primarily responsible for its resurgence later in the same century?
7. List the contraindications.

References

Brett H (1999) Aromatherapy in the care of older people. Nursing Times 95(33): 56–57.

Brown D (1993) Headway Guides: Aromatherapy. London: Hodder & Stoughton.

CHIPS (1996) The Chemical Hazardous Information and Packaging for Supply Regulations, Health and Safety Commission. London: HMSO.

COSHH (1994) The Control of Substances Hazardous to Health Regulations. London: HMSO.

Davis P (1999) Aromatherapy an A–Z, revised edn. Saffron Walden: CW Daniel Co. Ltd.

Fowler P, Wall M (1997) COSSH and CHIPS: ensuring the safety of aromatherapy. Complementary Therapies in Medicine 5: 112–115.

Fowler P, Wall M (1998) Aromatherapy, Control of Substances Hazardous to Health (COSHH) and assessment of the chemical risk. Complementary Therapies in Medicine 6: 85–93.

Franchomme P, Penoel D (1990) L'Aromatherapie Exactement. Limoges: Jollois.

Hopkins C (1995) Aromatherapy: Remedies for everyday ailments. Bristol: Parallel Books.

Jager W, Buchbauer G, Jirovetz, Fritzer M (1992) Percutaneous absorption of lavender oil from a massage oil. Journal of the Society of Cosmetic Chemists 43(1): 49–54 .

Mackereth P (1995) Aromatherapy – nice but not 'essential'. Complementary Therapies in Nursing and Midwifery 1: 4–7.

Mantle F (1999) NT Monographs. Complementary therapies: is there an evidence base? London: Emap Healthcare.

Maxwell-Hudson C (1988) The Complete Book of Massage. London: Dorling Kindersley Publishers Ltd.

Price S, Price L (1995) Aromatherapy for Health Professionals. Edinburgh: Churchill Livingstone.

Riley M, Foner A (1968) Aging and Society, Volume 1. New York: Trinity.

Stevensen C (1995) Aromatherapy. In: Rankin-Box D, ed., The Nurses' Handbook of Complementary Therapies. Edinburgh: Churchill Livingstone.

Tisserand R, Balacs T (1995) Essential Oil Safety: A guide for health care professionals. Edinburgh: Churchill Livingstone.

Valnet J (1990) The Practice of Aromatherapy. Saffron Walden: CW Daniel Co. Ltd.

Vickers A (1996) Massage and Aromatherapy: A guide for health professionals. London: Chapman & Hall.

Worwood V (1994) The Fragrant Pharmacy. London: Bantam Books.

CHAPTER 5

Reflexology (reflex zone therapy)

Reflexology is a therapy based on the theory that there are reflexes in the feet (and hands) that correspond to various parts of the body. By massaging these reflex areas in the feet and/or hands, reflexology aims to treat diseases in parts of the body that are said to be directly related to those areas or zones within the feet (and hands). The reflexes in the hands are deemed to be more difficult to access and less sensitive than those of the feet, so most reflexologists tend to use the feet in preference to the hands, unless there is a reason for the feet not be used.

Reflexology has been defined as:

> . . . a treatment which applies varying degrees of pressure to different parts of the body, usually the hands or feet, in order to promote health and well-being.
>
> Griffiths (1995)

Reflexology therefore aims to work with the body's own natural healing powers and create equilibrium and harmony within body, mind and spirit. Instead of suppressing these healing powers, it seeks to release and mobilise them so that they may help correct and maintain the body's natural balance and energy levels. It attempts to maintain this homoeostasis by regulating both over- and under-active systems. Not only is it a therapy to be used in times of illness, but it can also be effective in health promotion and disease prevention.

When Vickers (1996) reviewed the literature, however, he found little to recommend the use of reflexology, because he said that the few studies available to him were either flawed or inconclusive. Botting (1997) also reviewed the literature on reflexology treatments and noted that, although there was considerable anecdotal evidence to support their use as a therapy, she believed that much of it had been influenced by the beliefs and personal experiences of both the therapists and their patients. After examining some randomised controlled trials (RCTs), she stated that there was a paucity of good quality understandable research. She added that, although there were some foreign studies, often only part translations of this work were available. She therefore concluded, like Vickers (1996), that it was not easy to make accurate decisions about the efficacy of reflexology on such limited information.

Mackereth et al. (2000), however, felt that her work had seriously undermined people's belief in reflexology because she had not taken into account the fact that such practitioners incorporated into their care the best evidence available to them. They argued that:

> . . . anecdotal reports, practitioner reflections and single case studies [did] have a place in building experience and understanding [as they were] essential in identifying areas for more detailed and controlled research work.
>
> Mackereth et al. (2000)

They felt that, although it was unrealistic to expect all practitioners to become researchers, there was an onus on them to collect sound evidence about their practice. They believed that different opportunities were now 'opening up' to encourage this, and urged all involved in reflexology teaching and practice to share their special skills and, from that, to develop an informed, substantive, knowledge base together.

Historical background

Reflexology is regarded as a very ancient therapeutic treatment, yet its true origins remain unknown. It is said to have originated approximately 5000 years ago in China where practitioners stimulated pressure points and used them to correct imbalances in the patient's energy fields. It has been mooted that they did this to relieve pain. There is also evidence that in the fourth century BC Dr Wang-Wei was using it in conjunction with acupuncture. After positioning the acupuncture needles, he then applied very firm pressure to them with both his thumbs and the soles of his feet. He kept up the pressure until the desired effect was achieved because he maintained that it was this pressure that released the patient's healing potential. The ancient Indians and the Native Americans of North America were also both said to have practised reflexology. The latter are said still to be using it today in the same way as their forefathers. Other historical sources have speculated that the origins of reflexology began in the early Inca civilisations of Peru, dating back even further to 1200 BC.

Some feel, however, that it began in Egypt because of its depiction on a wall painting in the tomb of the physician Ankhmahor of Saqqara, south of Cairo, dating back to 2330 BC. This drawing shows two people being treated, one having foot massage and the other experiencing hand massage. Seemingly, it has been concluded that these treatments constituted reflexology. It is obvious, however, that the Chinese and Egyptians were practising and teaching similar things, and it has been postulated that the early Atlantean sailors may have ferried information between these two great cultures (Gillanders 1995)!

There is concrete evidence of its use by the Italian sculptor Benvenuto Cellini (1500–1571), who found that, if he exerted strong pressure on his fingers and toes, he experienced some pain relief. During the sixteenth century books on zone therapy began to appear in Europe. Dr Adamus and Dr A'tatis wrote the most notable text, published in 1582, but shortly afterwards Dr Ball published a similar work in Leipzig (Wills 1995). During the nineteenth century, the twentieth President of the USA, James Garfield (1831–1881), was reported to have used reflexology to help him recover from injuries sustained in an assassination attempt.

Modern reflexology

The leading proponent of modern-day reflexology appears to be Dr William Henry Fitzgerald (1872–1942), and most authors attribute reflexology to him. After graduating from Vermont University he worked as an ear, nose and throat (ENT) specialist in Boston City Hospital and then for a while in London and Vienna. He discovered his theory almost by accident while working in St Francis Hospital, Hartford, Connecticut. He noticed that patients experienced different levels of pain postoperatively and also that patients were unwittingly performing reflexology on themselves. When pressure was applied to specific parts of the hands and feet it caused some anaesthesia to corresponding areas in the body and:

> . . . would also bring about normal physiological action in all parts of the zone treated, no matter how remote this area may be from the part upon which the treatment is exerted.
>
> Ingham (1991)

On the basis of these findings he divided the body into 10 longitudinal zones (Figure 5.1). If you imagine a line drawn through the centre of the body from head to toe there will be five zones to the left and five to the right, e.g. zone 1 extends from the thumb to the big toe. The lines are, of course, not real and the zones (or segments) between them are all deemed

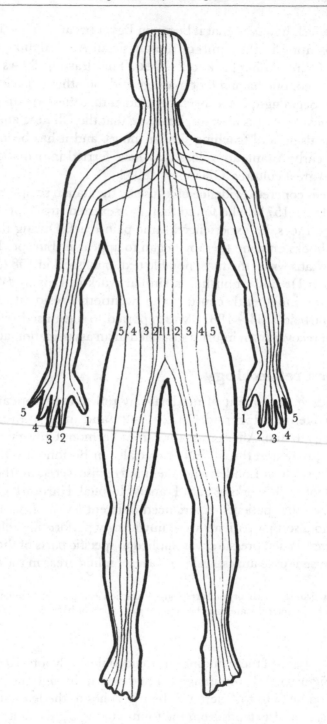

Figure 5.1 Diagrammatic representation of 10 longitudinal reflex zones.

to be equal in width. The importance is placed on the areas between the lines, as opposed to acupuncture and acupressure which treat the points on a designated meridian and collateral lines, because all parts of the body within each reflex zone are linked together, e.g. if there is a problem in one zone, it is likely that problems will be experienced in other parts of the same zone.

Fitzgerald used all sorts of instruments to test out his 'anaesthetic' theory by applying pressure to various parts of the body. He was said to have used clothes pegs, metal combs and elastic bands, and he thought the pressure should be applied for between 30 seconds and 5 minutes. He treated a wide range of disorders, such as headaches, eye and breathing disorders, and calculated his success rate at 75%. In 1917 he published with Dr Bowers entitled *Zone Therapy: Relieving pain at home.*

However, it was when he met Dr Joe Riley and his wife that his theories were given a much wider audience. They became interested and in turn influenced a young physiotherapist called Eunice Ingham (Stopfel), who further developed the theory in the 1930s. She developed a type of pressure massage and left her hospital post at St Petersburg, Florida, to set up in private practice as a reflexologist. Her work, the first book published on reflexology as we know it, published in 1938 (Ingham 1991), is still used by some therapists today. Unlike Fitzgerald she treated the body by concentrating only on the feet.

In the preface of her book, Ingham (1991) noted that during her practising years she and others established how:

> . . . each reflex and point of contact [was] carefully and thoughtfully checked and rechecked, until with all confidence we call your attention to these findings, sincerely trusting they will prove helpful and beneficial to others.
>
> Ingham (1991)

Before her death in 1974 she taught these skills to Doreen Baly, the person probably most responsible for encouraging the growth of modern reflexology in Britain. Baly (1988) who was also a qualified nurse, set up the first British training school in 1966.

Theories

It is not known exactly how reflexology works, although several theories abound. Tanner (1990) asserts that most therapists support the notion that the body is divided into 10 reflex zones or energy channels, which traverse the length of the body and extend into the feet. It is only when the energy flow is blocked that problems are thought to arise. There are many different schools of reflexology using varying techniques, but Griffiths (1995) asserted that the underlying principles of them are all similar.

Several theories have been mooted as to what happens and why during reflexology. Although there is a tremendous amount of anecdotal evidence to support these theories and several studies have been initiated to try to look at them, as yet no one theory has been clearly established. It has been suggested that crystalline deposits build up in the feet and cause problems within related organs. Ingham (1991) considered that these deposits of calcium and uric acid build up on the nerve endings of the feet as a result of bodily malfunction, and these in turn caused imbalance, tension or congestion in the whole of the affected zone. It is thought that, by applying massage to these zones, it will cause these deposits to disintegrate, be absorbed into the bloodstream and then be eliminated from the body, via the urine (Ingham 1991). They feel like grit or, as I prefer to say, granulated sugar under the skin. The nerve impulses are also stimulated to pass along the zones and they act to clear any congestion or blockage in these zones. Sahai (1993) stated that reflexology appears to act as a catalyst to healing as it:

... stimulates the body's self-regulatory and healing capability.

Sahai (1993)

Structure of the foot

The foot is a very complex structure and each foot is made up of 26 bones and 33 articulations. The posterior part of the foot contains the calcaneum and talus bones. The talus is the only bone that articulates with the fibula in the leg and during walking bears the entire weight of the body. Part of this weight is then transmitted to the largest and strongest bone of the foot, the calcaneum or heel bone, and the rest of the tarsal bones. The five metatarsal bones articulate with the first, second and third cuneiform and cuboid bones. The first metatarsal bone is the thickest of the bones and carries most weight. The metatarsals articulate with the phalanges.

There are two arches of the foot, the longitudinal (made up of medial and lateral aspects) and the transverse. These vary in size in different people. These arches provide leverage during walking and help support the weight of the body. Although the muscles in the foot are comparable to those in the hands, they are designed for support and locomotion. The hand muscles provide much more elaborate and accurate movements.

There are three transverse zones of each foot (see Figure 5.2 for a diagrammatic representation of the reflex and transverse zones of the soles of both feet). The first is where the metatarsals and phalanges meet, above the shoulder girdle line; the second at Lisfranc's joint line (where the metatarsals and tarsals meet), between the shoulder and waistline, and the third lies midway between the talus and calcaneum bones (including the malleoli), below the waistline and pelvic floor. Using the transverse zones and longitudinal zones together allows for a grid system to be built up, so that the reflex points can be more readily identified (Booth 1994). Lastly, in addition to these, there are 19 muscles, 107 ligaments and 72 000 nerve endings.

Mirror image

All the internal organs and bodily structures are said to be mirrored in the feet. There are many variations (see Figure 5.3 for diagrammatic representation of the major reflexes on the soles of both feet). The reflex points may vary from foot to foot. The charts must therefore act only as a guide to locate the various organs, glands and structures, but the general consensus for treatment is as follows:

1. Toes: head, brain, teeth, sinuses, sensory organs and upper lymphatics.
2. Between shoulder and waistline transverse zones: thoracic and upper abdominal organs and glands.
3. Between waistline and pelvic floor transverse zones: lower abdominal and pelvic organs and lower lymphatics.
4. Outer aspect of foot: all bony areas such as the shoulder, hip, knee and ankle.
5. Inner aspect of foot: spinal reflexes.

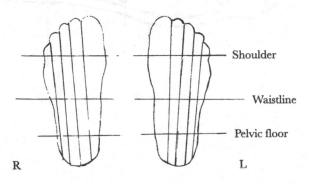

Figure 5.2 Diagrammatic representation of the reflex and transverse zones of both feet.

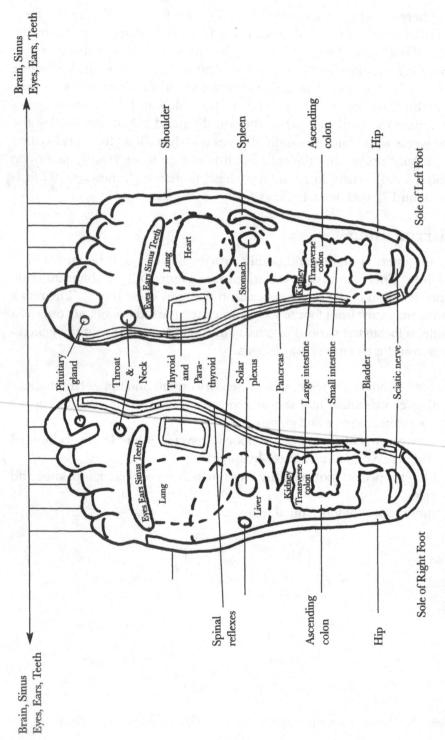

Figure 5.3 Diagrammatic representation of major reflexes on the soles of both feet.

There has been very little research into how bodily organs, etc. are actually mapped in the feet (or hands). Gillanders (1995) notes that a Japanese healer, Hiroshi Motoyama, studied the zones and electrically mapped the meridian endings in the fingers and toes. He found that when a meridian is blocked congestion occurs at this site, because of decreased energy flow. Omura (1994) also attempted to evaluate aspects of this. As there is such a wide variety of foot and hand charts used in different reflexology schools, Omura (1994) studied the accuracy of the most common ones. After mapping the organs using their specialist technique, he also found similar evidence to Motomaya and noted that even 1 minute of massage was likely to ease this congestion, give selective circulatory improvement and often ease pain. Omura's (1994) work also supported the notion that external abnormalities may influence reflex zone efficiency.

Advantages

- Non-invasive and harmless if used knowledgeably and intuitively.
- Inexpensive because no expensive equipment is required and it can be practised almost anywhere.
- Aids relaxation, calms and soothes, and may induce sleep and pain relief.
- Said to be particularly useful for relieving stress and tension conditions such as migraine and backache, asthma and allergies (Lynn 1996).
- Improves circulation of blood and lymph.
- Assists elimination of toxins, such as uric acid from the body.
- After massage healing powers are said to be released, to help correct and maintain harmonious balance in the body.
- Very few side effects and these are mostly of a transitory nature.
- Provides another type of touch.

Treatment

Abide by any protocols etc. that are in operation if you are using one within your care setting, obtain informed consent from the patient or another, and consider the following.

Environment

This should be warm, calm and private. Much of the advice about positioning that was given in Chapter 3 will apply. If a patient is unable to lie down easily, sit him or her in a chair and support both legs on a stool.

Always cover the lower limbs with a blanket to maintain modesty, because during treatment, when they relax, their legs may splay open. The patient should be bare foot and both feet should be placed on a towel and covered with another. It is not necessary to wash the patient's feet before treatment and indeed some therapists say that they should not because by so doing some of the clues to treatment would be lost. Some patients, however, feel uncomfortable about this. I find that non-medicated wet wipes are useful for freshening the feet.

Assessment

A full history should be taken and the patient's past and current problems should be noted on a record sheet such as that in Table 1.3. Alongside this, careful observation will be made.

Observation should be made of both feet

This needs to include both visual and manual observation to identify any abnormalities of skin, colour, shape, tissue, temperature, swelling, injury, conditions and also smell. It is essential to do this thoroughly because any abnormality is likely to cause a disturbance within the reflex zone affected. Abnormalities may include such things as: recent injury, inherited or congenital conditions, circulatory problems and arthritic toes. These must all be recorded and a simple addition to the assessment chart (Table 5.1) will facilitate this. I also find that if I draw an outline of both

Table 5.1 Foot record

	Right foot	Left foot
Colour		
Skin tone		
Hard skin		
Tissue viability		
Any lesions/bony deformities		
Skin conditions		
Skin temperature		
Swelling		
Muscle tone		
Flat foot		
High arch		
Odour		
Zone/area[a]		

[a]Here you will identify the zones and areas that require special attention.

feet I can highlight any abnormalities on it. This serves as a good pictorial record that is easy to compare with subsequent treatment records.

Post-treatment findings, including any reactions and all subsequent treatments, should be recorded on a continuation sheet and the pictorial foot chart, if using one.

Manual procedure

Before the exploratory part of the treatment may begin, the patient needs to feel relaxed and comfortable and the feet need to be warm. Do not use oil or talcum powder during the procedure because they will cause your hands to slip and you will not then be able to apply smooth and consistent pressure to the reflex zones.

1. Wash your hands.
2. Uncover both feet and cradle them in your hands. Now proceed with a series of relaxing movement. This allows time for the patient to get used to being touched and affords you an opportunity to gauge the exact pressure required. First perform slow and rhythmical effleurage (see Chapter 3), stroke firmly on the top of the foot from the toes to the ankle and continue with this on the underside of the foot back to the toes. Follow this with some gentle toe stretches. Hold each toe, in turn, gently between your finger and thumb and let your fingers slide from their ankle down to the tips of their toes. Rotate each toe twice in each direction. Then clasp and rotate the ankle clockwise and anti-clockwise. To finish off 'zig zag' down the sole of the foot from toes to heel with your thumbs Then hold the inner and outer edges of the patient's foot with both hands and manipulate it from side to side (this part of the procedure is very similar to that employed in the foot massage sequence in Chapter 3, but here you will not be using any oil). Finally make contact with the solar plexus (Figure 5.4) in both feet and encourage the patient to breathe in and out while you are doing this.
3. Once the patient is relaxed and used to this manual contact, begin the exploratory stage. Uncover one foot – normally the right foot – support it with one of your hands and with the other work systematically all over the foot using, what is affectionately called, a 'caterpillar walk', simply because it resembles the way a caterpillar moves! The caterpillar movement is performed by 'walking' your arched thumb or finger gently and rhythmically over the surface of the skin (see Figure 5.5 showing caterpillar walking along spinal reflexes). This must

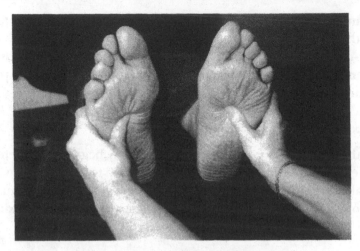

Figure 5.4 Making contact with the solar plexus of both feet.

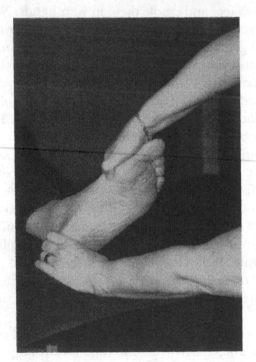

Figure 5.5 'Caterpillar walking' along some spinal reflexes in the left foot.

include not only the sole, but also the plantar and dorsal surfaces and the malleolus of each foot. You should always use the pad and never the tip of either your finger or your thumb. As they move, your finger or thumb will exert an even pressure on the minute reflex points under the skin.

Although you may treat the zones of the feet in any order, it is best to work in a logical and methodical way so that all of them are covered evenly. All areas should be treated so that you maintain harmony of the bodily organs. Having said that, if you detect any abnormalities, go over them again, but do not be tempted to over-treat and avoid those areas that are contraindicated. The pressure exerted will stimulate the reflex areas in the feet and this will encourage the nerve impulses to travel along the energy pathways to the parts of the body to which they connect. The pressure should be firm enough so that it does not tickle, but not so hard that it hurts. As the feet often feel rather sensitive at this time, some discomfort may be felt where there is a disorder in a particular reflex zone. Once the zone is harmonised, this discomfort should disappear. Patients say that it feels like the therapist is digging his or her nails into them. Figure 5.6 shows treating the upper lymphatics in the right foot and Figure 5.7 shows treating the head region of the left foot.

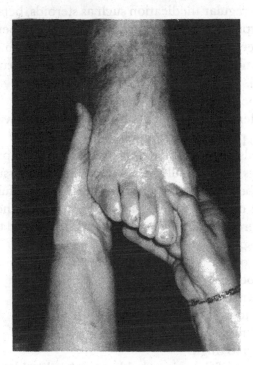

Figure 5.6 Treating the upper lymphatics on the right foot.

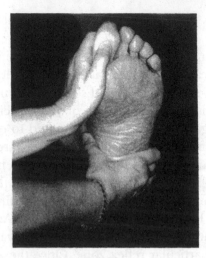

Figure 5.7 Treating the head region on the left foot.

Normal and healthy reflex zones are not painful to touch. Lett (1994) advises, however, that sensory perception may be heightened or reduced in the following:

– When on regular medication such as steroids, beta blockers, analgesics, hypnotics and tranquillisers, and while being treated with chemotherapy and radiotherapy. A lighter touch is required with these patients so that excretion of their drugs, etc. is not increased.

– During the dying process.

– In disorders of the central nervous and cardiovascular systems, psychosis, paralysis and vitamin deficiency.

You will also need to be extra careful over bony prominences, any abnormalities such as hallux valgus and any scar tissue, because they are likely to be painful. If a certain area is very painful, it is also useful to adopt the cross-reflex approach to treatment. The 'cross-reflexes' relate to different points on each side of the body and the following are said to correspond:

– shoulder to hip
– hand to foot
– ankle to wrist
– fingers to toes
– elbow to knee
– upper arm to thigh.

For instance, if there is a problem in the shoulder area, you could massage either both the shoulder and the knee areas or just the knee, its corresponding reflex, if the shoulder area was too painful. I liken this to the phenomenon of referred pain, e.g. after a cholecystectomy (removal of the gallbladder), referred pain is sometimes felt in the neck and upper shoulder area as well as in the site of the abdominal operation. For the patient to feel comfortable, both types of pain will need to be managed.

4. During treatment continue to use effleurage to soothe, relax and help eliminate toxins from the body.
5. Once the treatment is completed, cover the first foot and continue to treat the other foot in the same way. Remember that some of the points to cover are different from those in the first foot. Generally speaking, the organs of the right side of the body will be in the right foot and vice versa.
6. Uncover both feet and perform soothing and relaxing effleurage to both feet. For a few moments leave your hands on both feet so that the treatment does not end abruptly. It is said that this unites the body to make it whole once more.
7. Leave the patient to rest and wash your hands.
8. Documentation: evaluate the care given and make a note of the procedure adopted and any treatment outcomes in your records and/or foot chart. This is essential so that future treatments may be altered accordingly. Record any reactions.
9. Reactions: these might be experienced during or after treatment.

Reactions during a treatment

These include:

- A feeling of deep relaxation and the patient might even go to sleep.
- Muscular relaxation.
- Sighing, yawning and laughing.
- Sweating of the palms of their hands – this may indicate that the patient cannot tolerate any more treatment. I have also seen profuse sweating of the feet and lower limbs.

Reactions after and between treatments

These are very variable and may include:

- Deep relaxation
- Emotional changes
- Increased excretory action

- Skin reactions, good or bad
- Lethargy
- Feeling worse than before the treatment. It has been mooted that this occurs because, after reflexology, unresolved health problems may flare up, in the body's attempt to rebalance itself. Reflexologists do not view this negatively, because they believe that, in order to re-establish equilibrium and good health, underlying problems, as well as symptoms, need to be treated.

These feelings have been referred to as being part of a healing crisis and Sahai (1993) believed that they occurred as a result of the detoxification that occurs during and after a reflexology treatment.

Advice

Give adequate advice about the next treatment and for after the treatment, and without alarming him or her inform your patient about other reactions that might be experienced. Refer on if necessary.

Length and frequency of treatment

These will be dependent on the condition and needs of the patient, and whether it is a first or subsequent treatment. The average treatment tends to last between 20 and 30 min. Patients may require more than one or even several sessions before they experience any benefit from treatment. Treatments are normally performed no more than once or twice a week and if, after several sessions, no improvement is obvious, they should be evaluated and continued only if there is likely to be some future benefit, e.g. a terminally ill patient may continue to enjoy such treatment and, if no false claims are made or false hope given, it may be perfectly acceptable to continue because the benefit may be quite intangible (please see Chapter 14 for an example of where reflexology was given as an adjunct to the care of a dying patient).

Hand reflexology

This can be performed in much the same way as foot reflexology, but is said not to be so effective. It is particularly useful when a patient does not like his or her feet touched or when it is inadvisable to use them. Figure 5.8 gives a diagrammatic representation of the major reflexes on the palms of both hands; Figure 5.9 shows contacting the solar plexus with both hands and Figure 5.10 the 'caterpillar walk' in the right hand.

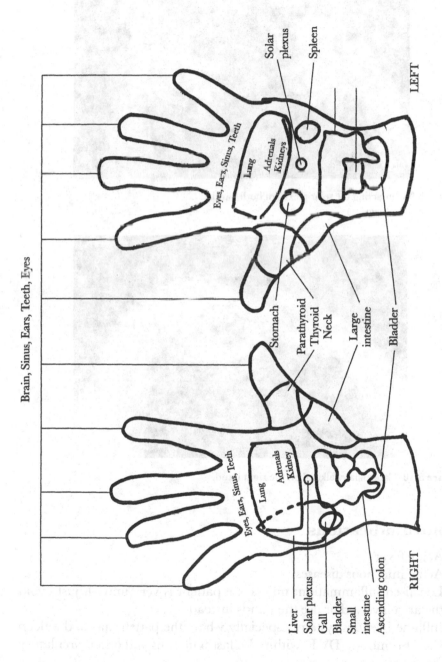

Figure 5.8 Diagrammatic representation of the major reflexes on the palms of both hands.

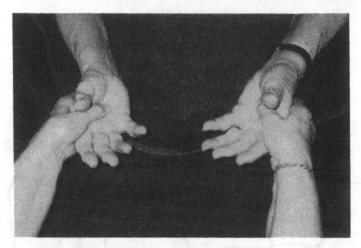

Figure 5.9 Contacting the solar plexus of both hands.

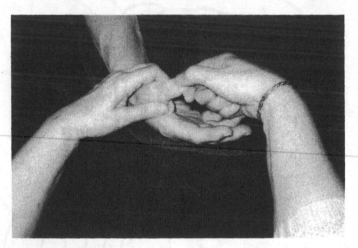

Figure 5.10 'Caterpillar walking' on the right hand.

Contraindications

- Acute fever
- Acute infectious diseases
- Localised inflammation: unless the patient is very unwell, just avoid the area involved or use the hands instead
- Inflamed venous system, especially where the patient has had a deep vein thrombosis (DVT) within the last 6 months and other circulatory disorders such as leg ulcers

- Acute and inflammatory conditions of the lymphatic system
- Intense and persistent or abnormal reactions during treatments
- When the patient's feet are severely infected or have suffered injury and burns
- After surgery.

Caution

Although reflexology may not be contraindicated in the following conditions, some caution is required:

- In the presence of kidney stones or gallstones because some therapists believe that the stones may be moved by the treatment and have the potential to cause an obstruction.
- For patients with pacemakers because pacemakers are also deemed to be able to be moved during treatment.

Combined treatments

Some practitioners who are qualified in several disciplines may combine compatible therapies in a single treatment. Using essential oils during a reflexology treatment is an example of this. I find that best results are obtained if I apply the essential oils, having diluted them first in a suitable carrier oil, directly to the reflex points themselves after the reflexology part of the treatment, e.g. cajuput (*Melaleuca leucadendron*) may be useful to apply to the head and lung area reflexes of a patient's feet who is already receiving reflexology for congestion.

In addition, it is quite acceptable to combine reflexology with flower remedies and Stormer (1995) gives many examples of this. I have found that using the Bach flower remedy, vervain (*Verbena officinalis*), alongside reflexology is very useful to promote sleep in anxious patients. This could be given orally or added to an oil and rubbed into the head and brain region. As well as this, with one very overwrought patient, I also added neroli bigarade (*Citrus aurantium*) because of its known antidepressant properties.

Please note that the same precautions will have to be taken as if you were giving an aromatherapy and/or flower remedy treatment, and your patient assessment must reflect this additional aspect of care. Remember that only those qualified or authorised to do so must initiate these treatments. (Please see Chapters 4 for guidance on the use of aromatherapy and Chapter 6 for flower remedies.)

Reflexology does appear to have a place in the treatment of older adults and seems most suitable for help with chronic conditions. Many claims have been made about its efficacy in the treatment of many different conditions, but some caution must be exercised over this. Nurses are now attempting to build up a substantive therapeutic knowledge base and are increasingly keen to practise it, especially as more and more patients appear to be interested in it. Therefore, as a complementary therapy it may, if developed strategically, have the potential to enhance emotional and physical well-being.

Questions

Try to answer the following:

* What is reflexology and what are its main theories?
* Briefly describe the major stages in the historical development of reflexology.
* How will you perform reflexology and what is the significance of the cross-reflexes?
* When making an oral and visual patient assessment, before treatment, what would you particularly look for and why?
* Who might benefit from reflexology and why?
* Identify the contraindications to reflexology.
* When would you perform reflexology on the hands in preference to the feet?

References

Baly D (1988) Reflexology Today. Vermont: Healing Arts Press.

Booth B (1994) Reflexology. Nursing Times 90(1): 38–140.

Botting D (1997) Review of literature on the effectiveness of reflexology. Complementary Therapies in Nursing and Midwifery 3: 123–130.

Gillanders A (1995) Reflexology: A step-by-step guide. London: Gaia Books Ltd.

Griffiths P (1995) Reflexology. In: Rankin-Box D, ed., The Nurses' Handbook of Complementary Therapies. Edinburgh: Churchill Livingstone .

Griffiths P (1996) Reflexology. Complementary Therapies in Nursing and Midwifery 2: 13–16.

Ingham E (1991) The original works of Eunice D. Ingham. Stories the feet can tell thru reflexology – Stories the feet have told thru reflexology (with revisions by Dwight C. Byers). St Petersburg, FL: Ingham Publishing, Inc.

Lett A (1994) Reflex zone therapy. In: Wells R, Tschudin V, eds, Wells' Supportive Therapies in Health Care. London: Baillière Tindall.

Lynn J (1996) Using complementary therapies: reflexology. Professional Nurse 11(5): 321–322.

Mackereth P, Dryden S, Frankel B (2000) Reflexology: recent research approaches. Complementary Therapies in Nursing and Midwifery 6: 66–71.

Omura Y (1994) Accurate localization of organ representation areas on the feet and hands using the bi-digital O-ring test resonance phenomenon: its clinical diagnosis and treatment. 1. Acupuncture and Electro-Therapeutics Research 19(2–3): 153–190.

Sahai I (1993) Reflexology – its place in modern healthcare. Professional Nurse August: 722–725.

Stormer C (1995) Reflexology. The Definitive Guide. Reading: Hodder & Stoughton.

Tanner R (1990) Step by Step Reflexology. Surrey: Douglas Barry.

Vickers A (1996) Massage and Aromatherapy: A guide for health professionals. London: Chapman & Hall.

Wills P (1995) The Reflexology Manual. Hong Kong: Eddison Sadd Editions.

CHAPTER 6
Flower remedies

The use of flowers for healing the emotions is not new. The Ancient Egyptians and Australian Aboriginal people used them centuries ago. They were also popular in the Middle Ages, and there are examples of writings in the fifteenth century explaining how dew was collected from plants and used to treat imbalances. Such use of flowers for health purposes follows traditional as opposed to orthodox medical philosophies and Dr Edward Bach (pronounced Batch) rediscovered their potential for healing in the 1930s.

Dr Edward Bach (1886–1936)

Bach was an orthodox medical practitioner who had become disillusioned with the practice of only treating primarily physical symptoms. As a result of this he eventually gave up his lucrative practice in 1930 so that he could develop a total system of remedies that would combat all negative states of mind. He was convinced that it was these that adversely influenced healing. His work was also greatly influenced by his own feelings because he often experienced inner disharmony before finding the appropriate flower with which to make the remedy. He wrote:

> Disease is in essence the result of conflict between the Soul and the Mind, and will never be eradicated except by spiritual and mental effort. Such efforts, if properly made with understanding ... can cure and prevent disease by removing those basic factors, which are its primary cause. No effort directed to the body alone can do more than superficially repair damage, and in this, there is no cure, since the cause is still operative, and may at any moment again demonstrate its presence in another form ...
>
> Let it be briefly stated that disease, though apparent so cruelly, is in itself beneficent and for our own good, and if rightly interpreted, will guide us to our essential faults .... Suffering is a corrective to point out a lesson which by other means we have failed to grasp, and never can be eradicated until that lesson is learnt.
>
> Bach (1973)

He died shortly after he had identified the 38 remedies and the composite Rescue Remedy in 1936. It was said that he had died happy in the knowledge that he had achieved what he had set out to do (Anon 1995). The following list provides only a very brief insight into the key symptoms (Scheffer 1990) associated with each of the remedies and are grouped together under seven major categories identified by Bach (Rudd 1998). Further explanation can be found in Howard (1990).

Apprehension (fear)

Aspen (*Populus tremula*): for unknown fear, that may occur suddenly and for no apparent reason. Contrasts with mimulus.

Cherry plum (*Prunus cerasifera*): for those who experience irrational and desperate thoughts.

Mimulus (*Mimulus guttatus*): for those who are fearful of known things such as living alone, illness or death.

Red chestnut (*Aesculus carnea*): for those who are overly concerned and fearful for others.

Rock rose (*Helianthemum nummularium*): for those who experience terror after an unpleasant incident. This is usually a brief episode related to a particular event. This remedy also helps nightmares.

Loneliness

Heather (*Calluna vulgaris*): for self-obsessed people, sometimes hypochondriacs, who need to be constantly listened to. Such people are often shunned.

Impatiens (*Impatiens glandulifera*): for nervy, impatient people who do not 'suffer fools gladly'.

Water violet (*Hottonia palustris*): for proud, reserved, sensitive people with a tendency to become withdrawn.

Insufficient interest in present circumstances

Chestnut bud (*Aesculus hippocastanum*): for those who are unable to learn by and continually perpetuate their mistakes in both personal and professional relationships.

Clematis (*Clematis vitalba*): for preoccupied and often discontented people who yearn for a better life, yet tend to do little to achieve this.

Honeysuckle (*Lonicera caprifolium*): for those who are unable to 'move on' in their lives and seek solace in living in the past, e.g. homesickness and bereavement. Useful to combine with walnut.

Mustard (*Sinapsis arvensis*): for those who are suddenly depressed for no apparent reason.

Olive (*Olea europaea*): for those who are both physically and emotionally exhausted.

White chestnut (*Aesculus hippocastanum*): for those who are preoccupied by persistent worry that causes them to lack concentration and have difficulty sleeping.

Wild rose (*Rosa canina*): for those resigned, apathetic and over-accepting of their situation and who are therefore unable to attain their real potential.

Oversensitive to ideas and influence

Agrimony (*Agrimonia eupatoria*): for those who appear outwardly happy and content but are inwardly worried.

Centaury (*Centaurium umbellatum*): for weak people who are unable to say no and consequently become overburdened and have little time for themselves. Very useful for carers.

Holly (*Ilex aquifolium*): for those who feel anger, hatred, envy, jealousy, resentment and malice. It may go undetected because people tend to hide these emotions. It must be differentiated from willow.

Walnut (*Juglans regia*): for those who need to be assisted to 'move on' in their lives after a period of change such as puberty, the menopause, divorce, or obtaining a new house or job. Useful to combine with honeysuckle.

Despondency and despair

Crab apple (*Malus pumila*): for those who feel 'unclean' and require 'cleansing'. They may be ashamed and even disgusted by an aspect of their life.

Elm (*Ulmus procera*): for able people who temporarily feel inadequate and overwhelmed by their current responsibilities.

Larch (*Larix decidua*): for those lacking in self-confidence who feel inferior and sure to fail.

Oak (*Quercus robur*): for those who are normally strong over-achieving individuals who no longer feel able to struggle on.

Pine (*Pinus sylvestris*): for those who constantly apologise and blame themselves even for mistakes made by others.

Star of Bethlehem (*Ornithogalum umbellatum*): for those who have suffered mental, physical and emotional trauma and need help, immediately or much later, so that they may cope with the aftermath.

Sweet chestnut (*Castanea sativa*): for those experiencing utter dejection and inconsolable sorrow that may follow years of struggle or bereavement.

Willow (*Salix vitellina*): for those who abdicate responsibility for their lives and feel very 'hard done by'. They take on an almost martyred air and appear to gain some pleasure from their discontent.

Over-caring about the welfare of others

Beech (*Fagus sylvatica*): for intolerant and uncompromising people who constantly criticise others.

Chicory (*Cichorium intybus*): for manipulative, domineering and somewhat interfering individuals, especially when caring for their own.

Rock water (*Aqua petra*): for those who are opinionated, rigid and self-denying. Such individuals also tend to be dissatisfied with their own performance.

Vervain (*Verbena officinalis*): for intransigent, highly achieving, strong-willed individuals who may be unable to relax or sleep easily.

Vine (*Vitis vinifera*): for ambitious, domineering, autocratic, arrogant bullies who tend to override other people's wishes.

Uncertainty

Cerato (*Ceratostigma willmottiana*): for self-doubters who constantly ask others for advice even though they are perfectly able to make their own decisions.

Gentian (*Gentiana amarella*): for easily discouraged and depressed people when things are difficult.

Gorse (*Ulex europaeus*): for extremely despondent and pessimistic people who have almost given up, especially after experiencing chronic illness and inadequate treatments.

Hornbeam (*Carpinus betulus*): for those who doubt their ability to face the day ahead.

Scleranthus (*Scleranthus annus*): for indecisive people who are unable to make clear choices.

Wild oat (*Bromus ramosus*): for those who are unfulfilled and unable to make important decisions, especially about their future.

The composite Rescue Remedy, used in emergency situations, will be discussed later in the chapter.

The making of the remedies

Although 37 of the above remedies were prepared from tree blossoms and wild flowers, rock water was made from water from a natural spring that Bach thought contained therapeutic properties. To make the remedies he either floated the blossoms and flowers in a bowl of water and left them in the sunshine because sunrays are said to bring energy to the water (Mantle 1997) or lightly boiled them. In both methods he used brandy to preserve them. After diluting the essences twice, they were bottled for both stock and individual use. The resulting essences are so dilute that any direct chemical effect is considered to be negligible.

Mode of action

Although the rationale behind their action is unclear, it is hypothesised that the remedies work by resonating with some higher order. Scheffer (1990, pages 24–25) explains Bach's sentiments in this way:

> Bach said that the flower essences establish direct contact with the Higher Self of the Personality and thus become active in all aspects of our nature, in all parts of the aura. The planes of the aura are not subject to the laws of space and time which the physical body has to follow, and incipient illness can therefore be healed even before it shows itself in the physical body . . . . The Bach Flower Remedies (therefore) enter into direct contact with the Higher Self of Man . . . and act as divine energy impulses, across all energy levels.
>
> Scheffer (1990)

Although the above concepts are very hard to understand, there does seem to be some evidence, albeit anecdotal, that the remedies are useful (Mantle 1997). Instead of spending many hours attempting to unravel some of these theoretical complexities, it may be useful initially to think of them as agents that have the potential to act as catalysts for healing.

Selection and dosage

The Bach flower remedies can be taken internally even by very old people with no known side effects because it is claimed that they are neither toxic nor habit forming. So far there have been no clinical trials conducted on their use that can firmly substantiate this (Mantle 1997, Howard 1998). As the remedies are deemed to work on the individual's negative thought processes, it is essential to assess the patient's total condition (not just his or her symptoms) accurately so that the most appropriate remedy may be chosen. With such a vast array to choose from, it is tempting to feel that your patient or even you may need them all. You could liken this phenomenon to when you opened a medical textbook for the first time and were convinced that you had most of the diseases listed within it!

Do resist this and pick a combination of essences that are the most suitable. You will therefore need to use a selection that covers all facets of the patient's mental and emotional state. Some therapists are aided in this by the use of a pendulum because diagnosis is supposed to be made by an instinctual rather than intellectual process. I personally am not very adept at this and rely more heavily on what the patient does and does not say.

The remedies are very useful as an adjunct to other therapies and examples of this are given in later chapters. To be able to use these remedies effectively you need to be 'in tune' not only with your patients' emotional needs but also your own because Scheffer (1990) asserts that, if your own life and relationships are chaotic, it is difficult to help others heal their disharmonies. It would seem that these flower essences are not 'remedies' in the true sense because their aim is not to treat an external cause of disease but rather to redirect our life's energy into balance and thus '. . . energize our own health processes without unduly interfering in its natural flow' (Bach 1973).

When choosing the flower remedies, one to three are normally deemed sufficient to deal with the patient's negative states. Using too many together may actually muddle the procedure, but if you inadvertently choose the wrong one it is not harmful As the patient's emotional needs change different remedies may be introduced. As this is primarily a self-help therapy, the onus of healing rests with the patient rather than the therapist.

Dosage

The remedies may be taken singly, dropped straight onto the tongue, neat from the stock bottle (readily available from most health food stores) or in a glass of water. Bach advocated 4 drops four times per day. If using a combination of drops it is advisable to make up a solution. The easiest way to do this is to drop the chosen remedies into a 30 ml dropper bottle from the stock bottles, add 25 ml of pure spring water and one teaspoon of brandy to act as a preservative, then label clearly with the patient's name and dosage instructions. This would normally be 4 drops onto the tongue four to six times daily. As the remedies can also be used externally, if the patients prefer, up to 6 drops could be added to their bath or 2 drops to their massage oil. I, like Stormer (1995), also combine them with my reflexology treatments.

Having outlined the key elements associated with all of the above remedies, I would like now to introduce you to 10 remedies that I, personally, think are valuable to use with older people and their carers. The remedies are not a panacea for all ills, but may act as a liberating force for healing.

Aspen

This is often called the 'trembling tree' because its silver leaves appear to move and shimmer in the gentle wind. Aspen aims to elicit fearlessness and encourage patients to look more openly at their individual experiences. Aspen types are often fearful for no apparent reason and do not even know why this is. Their fear may occur suddenly, be accompanied by anxiety, apprehension and even trepidation, and evoke non-specific or vague irrational and disconcerting feelings of panic. They may experience nightmares or wake up terrified to go back to sleep in case these mental images return and they may also dwell unnecessarily on thoughts of death and dying. They appear to be stuck in a recurring cycle of fearing from which they cannot escape.

Aspen, as opposed to mimulus, helps individuals to get their fear into perspective because it gives them the courage not only to cope with their fears but also to address any arising conflicts. It also has the potential to act as a reassuring agent so that in time such individuals are able to balance the negative with the positive and become more realistic in their worrying. In addition, it is said to benefit both abusers of alcohol and those who have concerns about regular drug taking (not necessarily illegally) (Scheffer 1990).

Centaury

The annual centaury is associated with self-determination and self-realisation (Scheffer 1990) and its essence is especially considered valuable for weak-willed, passive, exploited or imposed upon people. It is therefore excellent for carers who need to learn to say no, especially those who find it hard to stand up to the emotional and physical demands of another. These carers tend to be kindly but also overly protective of their patients, and do not realise that they also need time for themselves. They may become ill or stressed because they often give more of themselves than they should but they fear confrontation. They are often very dissatisfied about this behaviour but are genuinely unable to alter it (Anon 1995).

Centaury affords protection for such people because it elicits inner strength and gives direction to what they can realistically accomplish. It helps them lose their 'doormat' mentality and become self-assertive, without being aggressive. After a time such individuals are able to express their own needs and identify priorities unimpeded by others. More importantly, however, it encourages gentle, kindly people to be forceful while letting them retain those caring qualities that they so value (Howard 1990).

Cherry plum

The cherry plum relates to openness and composure (Scheffer 1990) and appears to be essential for the deeply despairing. Such individuals are dreadfully afraid that they are 'going mad', are often depressed and may even be suicidal. These attacks may be both acute and chronic and they may require much more help than this remedy alone can provide. They tend to be highly strung, overly anxious people who at times may be hysterical or violent. This remedy can act only as a support to the other interventions that they most surely require, but it is useful to help these people regain their composure and find courage and inner strength to go on.

Crab apple

This acts as a very powerful cleanser and is especially beneficial for those who are experiencing self-disgust and loathing. They may feel either mentally or physically revolted and ashamed of a disease from which they are suffering, such as cancer, a skin disorder or AIDS. Such hypersensitive individuals are said to be perfectionists and find great difficulty in dealing with what lies ahead of them. They are also openly nervous of any environmental contaminants and are often intolerant of the attempts of others to help them. As a result of this they may become obsessional about cleansing routines.

It has been noted (Anon 1995) that everyone could benefit from this remedy because to a greater or lesser extent we all have some self-loathing. It is particularly useful for helping individuals control these irrational thoughts and start to see them in their proper perspective. Once they become more accepting, they can then begin to alter their own attitudes towards them. It goes well with the cleansing, essential oil juniper (*Juniperus communis*) to assist inner and outer cleansing.

Gorse

Gorse symbolises hope and is particularly useful for those who are despairing. Such people are extremely pessimistic, defeatist and have given up all hope for the future. These traits can be seen in patients suffering from chronic and terminal conditions, especially where they have either been subjected to a variety of unsuccessful treatments or have been told that their condition is incurable. Although they may not always feel utterly hopeless, they tend to feel condemned to a future of intolerable pain and suffering and so choose to 'give up'.

This remedy, as opposed to wild rose, can lift their spirits and help them to realise that being very negative will not help their condition. Although it is important that these individuals are not given false hope, some reasonable hope may help them cope with their current burden. It could help them to have more realistic expectations of and endure any palliative care more positively. It might even give them the strength to refuse further treatment.

Honeysuckle

This fragrant climbing shrub is vital for those who miss out on life because they constantly hark back to the past. Such individuals have little or no interest in current events and use past memories as an escape route from reality. These feelings often manifest after a bereavement or when leaving their own homes, perhaps to enter an institution. Although it is normal to value their past lives and memories, these people are often overly nostalgic and are unable to adapt to change. Sometimes thoughts of getting older make people react in this way.

Honeysuckle has the potential to help them to remember their memories lovingly without allowing them to dominate the future. They are also able to value and learn from past events but are at the same time encouraged to 'move on' and be more accepting of current times (Scheffer 1990). It is useful to combine with walnut to aid transitional change or with star of Bethlehem where there is unresolved sorrow, grief or shock.

Impatiens

This fleshy annual embodies patience and gentleness, and is particularly recommended for those who are nervously frustrated, as opposed to vervain, which is useful for inner tension (Scheffer 1990). Impatiens types, as the name suggests, are impatient and irritable, anger quickly and are often intolerant. They do not 'suffer fools gladly' and expect perfection. Such people make unpopular managers because they tend to be somewhat self-willed, would rather not delegate tasks and are easily irritated by mistakes made by inexperienced junior staff. Consequently, they do not make good team players, and often come to this role rather reluctantly. Impatiens is likely to be beneficial to such people because it helps them to be not only patient and tactful with their subordinates, but also more empathetic towards them. The essential oil Roman chamomile (*Anthemis nobilis*) goes well with this remedy.

Larch

This graceful tree is associated with self-confidence and therefore of particular value for those who are self-doubting (Anon 1995). These individuals lack self-confidence, are indecisive and are convinced that they are inferior to others. Although they secretly recognise that they are very able and have the potential to succeed, they do nothing about it in case they fail. Even though they admire success, their inability to rise to a challenge curtails their own professional and personal openings.

Larch, as opposed to cerato, can act as a prop and give negative individuals the courage both to confront and to embrace new opportunities creatively. As you may imagine, it could benefit the acutely ill, those in long-term and rehabilitative care, the abused or sexually impotent, and even carers because it encourages more objectivity in self-assessment of need. It can be combined with centaury for those who allow themselves to be treated as 'doormats'.

Mimulus

This yellow flowered perennial is associated with courage and confidence (Scheffer 1990) and is especially useful for those who are aware of their fears and the reasons behind them. Sufferers may be fearful of many things such as living alone, impending death or terminal disease. These fears, temporary or longer term, may be their own or related to close friends and dependants. Although some individuals inevitably, over time, adjust to such fears and worries and become less aware of their problems, others continue to find the challenges of daily life overwhelming.

Mimulus types are characteristically talented, shy and reserved, yet may come across as extroverts in their attempt to cover up their nervousness. They tire and sicken easily and often feel burdened. Mimulus, as opposed to aspen or rock rose, gives courage to those trying to overcome their fears. It allows people to be more assertive and self-protective. It is said that once individuals take mimulus they set in motion a process that helps develop more positive attitudes towards life's pressures. As this process continues, they start to view their difficulties as challenges to be conquered. This, in turn, leads on to a greater self-awareness and the realisation that it is not the problem itself that is hurting them but their attitude towards it. This liberation from such habituated behaviour has been likened to a 'healing crisis,' and regarded as the first step to recovery. Although this essence may not eradicate all feelings of fear, it enables them to deal with each experience.

Olive

This is one of the most valuable of the remedies and relates to 'the principle of regeneration, peace and restored balance' (Scheffer 1990). It acts as a calming agent for those who are fatigued, exhausted and drained of energy. This could be because they are wracked by disease, are enduring lengthy treatments, recuperating from illness or just involved in the process of caring for an invalid. To cope with these things, they have used all their inner reserves and are functioning very much below par. This mental or physical exhaustion may be either temporary or long term, but classically such sufferers present as a spent force who are too tired to carry on.

Olive is valuable to us all because it revives and replenishes depleted energy stocks. Its action encourages individuals to listen to their own needs, get 'in tune' with their own body and then pace their resultant activities accordingly. Once those afflicted have greater peace of mind and more vitality, the easier it should be for them to cope with further onslaughts.

Walnut

Walnut is particularly useful for those who are experiencing major changes such as moving home or the menopause and need help to adjust. The situation may be only temporary but vacillating, sensitive people seem to be those most affected. Such individuals' powers of decision-making at these times may be adversely influenced, not only by others, but also by their own self-imposed restrictions.

This remedy gives constancy and protection, the freedom from limiting influences and the chance to rethink one's whole approach to life. By also endowing protection against domineering personalities, past practices and events, it offers opportunities to shed irrational fears, break with past ties and 'move on' in our lives with courage. The essential oil cypress (*Cupressus sempervirens*) may also help this process.

Rescue Remedy

Perhaps this is the most well-known and widely used of all the remedies. This all-purpose, composite remedy is made up of star of Bethlehem, rock rose, impatiens, cherry plum and clematis (please see individual remedies for their specific action). As its name suggests, it is beneficial for those involved in real or perceived emergency situations because it acts to ameliorate the effects of any fear, anguish, panic or shock that may manifest. Scheffer (1990) gives various examples of how this remedy has even saved lives while victims awaited professional help. In distressing situations, it therefore provides comfort and reassurance and also has the ability to elicit calmness in those confounded by such torment. In addition, it is said to centre and ground an individual during periods of extreme stress or trauma.

It is inadvisable to use this remedy routinely because this might render it ineffective in times of urgent need. It would be preferable to keep it for purely emergency situations so that you do not become immune to its therapeutic effects. In acute situations 4 drops, from the stock bottle, are added to a glass of water and sipped slowly until the shocked feelings subside. If there is no water available, the patient is unconscious or should not drink, the remedy may be applied externally to the temples, back of the neck or both wrists, and repeated as necessary. Rescue Remedy is also available as a cream.

Foreign essences

As people travel extensively these days, it is valuable to consider some of the remedies now available from further afield.

Australian remedies

I first became interested in these essences when I had the opportunity to discuss their efficacy with therapists on a recent Australian visit.

Bush flower essences

Australia is a relatively unpolluted land and has the world's oldest and highest number of flowering plants available. Partly because of this, the herbalist and naturopath Ian White developed the Bush flower essences. He identified 62 specific remedies, which he developed from native flowers. He advocated that they should be used as a catalyst to rid us of our negative beliefs and thus boost our own healing potential. Although he recognised the worth of the Bach flower remedies, he felt that there was a need to create essences that could help people with more modern-day concerns such as sexuality, communication issues and spiritual need. The essences are used in much the same way as the Bach flower remedies, and are said to be particularly useful in helping us gain insight into our own problems, which then enables us to strengthen our pursuit of our life's goals. It is felt that the more we use them the more adept we become at ridding ourselves of our negative emotions. When we achieve this and are more positive in our thinking, equilibrium is re-established. Hakansan (1998) notes that they are used in this way within current Aboriginal culture to help them confront and resolve the difficulties of the day. In addition to this, some Aboriginal tribes also use them to help them make sense of their ancient stories (dreamings) and thus understand even more of their rich past heritage.

Some of the essences have wonderful names:

- Kangaroo Paw which is used for self-centred people who are insensitive to the needs of others
- Old Man Banksia which helps people cope with life's surprises
- Billy Goat Plum which is useful for people who are ashamed or even disgusted by their own body.

There are also 14 composite remedies available. The following selection is used: to help one travel; to harmonise hormonal imbalance; to enhance confidence and energy; and to deal with a perceived emergency. The recommended dosage is 7 drops twice daily and these are administered directly into the mouth from the stock bottle. They are used for a maximum of 2 weeks at a time. If the problem has not been resolved, they may be repeated or a different essence selected.

Western Australian flower essences

These are uniquely produced from the flowering plants of Western Australia. Two doctors, V and K Barneo, discovered them while working with an Aboriginal community who were using them (Balinski 1998). These people had continued to make these traditional remedies from recipes that supposedly dated back 40 000 years. Flowers are collected and left immersed in a clear glass container for a few hours in the sun. Once the flowers are discarded, the remaining stored water becomes the essence.

Although the underpinning philosophy of using these essences to balance the emotional state of an individual is similar to both the Bush flower and Bach flower systems, their usage is different. The chosen remedies are applied either to identified floral acupoints or to areas of the body that are painful. As a result of this Balinski (1998) notes how useful they are as an adjunct to other touch therapies, and gives examples of how she has used various remedies in conjunction with massage to assist pain and stress management, fatigue and postoperative shock.

There are many other essences around the world and possibly the most well known of these is the Californian poppy essence. Richard Katz made this originally in the 1970s. Although he had extensively used the Bach flower remedies, he also recognised that in North America there were also many beautiful plants with healing potential. Currently the Flower Essence Society currently produce 103 essences and are continuing to develop others (Rudd 1998).

Flower remedies are becoming increasingly popular and appear to have a place in the emotional care of older patients. If used with caution, they are safe and are deemed to have the potential to act as a catalyst for healing.

Questions

Try to answer the following questions, using the above information:

1. A patient wakes, panic stricken, for no apparent reason in the night and is afraid to go back to sleep. What remedy will you choose and why?
2. You notice that a member of staff is very intolerant and does not 'suffer fools gladly'. Why might he or she benefit from impatiens?
3. A recently widowed woman enters a nursing home and is very sad at leaving behind her home with all its memories. Why might the combination of walnut and honeysuckle help her? Would there be any benefit in adding star of Bethlehem to this solution?
4. How is Rescue Remedy different from the other Bach flower remedies and when would you use it?
5. Carefully select no more than three remedies that you think would be beneficial to you. How have you reached this decision?

References

Anon (1995) The Work of Dr Edward Bach: An introduction and guide to the 38 Flower Remedies. London: Wigmore Publications Ltd.

Bach E (1973) Heal Thyself. Oxford: CW Daniel Co. Ltd.

Balinski A (1998) Use of Western Australian flower essences in the management of pain and stress in the hospital setting. Complementary Therapies in Nursing and Midwifery 4: 111–117.

Brown D (1993) Headway Lifeguides. Massage. London: Hodder & Stoughton

Hakanson D (1998) Oracle of the Dreamtime. Aboriginal Dreamings offer guidance for today. London: Connections Book Publishing Ltd.

Howard J (1990) The Bach Flower Remedies Step by Step. Saffron Walden: CW Daniel Co. Ltd.

Howard J (1998) Bach Flower Remedies: a personal commentary on the work of Dr Edward Bach. Complementary Therapies in Nursing and Midwifery 4: 148–149.

Mantle F (1997) Bach flower remedies. Complementary Therapies in Nursing and Midwifery 3: 142–144.

Rudd C (1998) Flower Essences: An illustrated guide. Shaftesbury, Dorset: Element Books Ltd.

Scheffer M (1990) Bach Flower Therapy. Theory and practice. London: Thorsons.

Stormer C (1995) Reflexology. The definitive guide. London: Hodder & Stoughton Educational.

Application to practice

For this part I have adopted an interactive approach to encourage you to question the therapies chosen, their supporting rationale and the means by which you may be able to take them forward in the care of older people. Some of the information presented is inevitably anecdotal.

The case studies

Although all the patients who kindly agreed to be used as case study examples were managed individually, there were elements of their care that was the same. To avoid repetition within the following chapters, I have included them here. To uphold confidentiality pseudonyms are used and no reference is given to any personal details that might identify them. Fully informed consent was obtained from either the patient or the appropriate person and privacy was assured at all times. On the initial visit a full oral and visual assessment was made and documented, and at subsequent visits patient progress was evaluated and treatment restructured accordingly. I involved the patient and/or carer in each consultation as much as possible and some quiet time was encouraged afterwards.

The case studies will not only be disease and therapy specific but will also show where therapies may usefully be combined. The examples given draw heavily not only from my own and other practitioners' experiences, but also from research-based evidence.

Please note that it is essential to have any underlying causes of disease thoroughly investigated before treating any symptoms. Remember also that only an appropriately qualified person or someone who has been approved and authorised to practise a delegated task should carry out these interventions.

Part III

Application to practice

CHAPTER 7

The mental, emotional and neurological state

As the nervous system is the major communication system of the body, if there is a breakdown or slowing of it, the body will work less efficiently From the age of 25, it has been estimated that there is a gradual and steady loss of neurons, but function is mostly sustained and it may be that the losses occur in the central nervous system (CNS) because older people either need or use fewer of these circuits. It seems that the central, parasympathetic and autonomic nervous systems are all affected by ageing, but the extent of their decline varies within individuals, which are therefore likely to influence homoeostasis adversely. These losses do not, however, necessarily correlate to the amount of problems that a patient may display as, for instance, some individuals with reduced brain capacity will display little or no significant symptoms whereas others with normal brain capacity may show impaired performance.

Stereotypes suggest that a high proportion of older people experience mental health problems, but this is a fallacy. In fact, most cope very well with the changes and inevitable losses associated with ageing and only a small minority is seriously affected (Norman 1992). One must remember that old age is a very individual and subjective experience that is strongly influenced by our past lives and future emotional well-being and appears to be dependent on maintaining some normality of living at this time. As a result of the onset of physical ill-health, however, this may be compromised, especially where personal independence is at risk.

Although individuals perceive this differently and mental health problems are not an inevitable consequence of ageing, it is generally thought that it is this deterioration that exacerbates dissatisfaction. This is also affected by social and economic influences, which cannot be considered here. When treating such patients, it is therefore very important to recognise this link between physical and mental processes and treat both. This

119

will rely on the use of good assessment techniques and the formalisation of appropriate and realistic interventions, which aim to encourage patient individuality and maximise their functional and activity levels. To do this, the emphasis may be on the management of their physical symptoms, although, in all cases, treatment must not further exacerbate any confusion or disorientation that may be present. The achievement of effective complementary therapy will be more likely if you work closely not only with the patient but also with their formal and informal carers, especially if you have only a limited knowledge of such patients and their conditions.

There is much anecdotal evidence but hardly any published studies to support the use of complementary therapies in mental health. There is, however, limited evidence that they are used successfully with people with learning, emotional and behavioural difficulties. Vickers (1996) in his review notes that:

> . . . the role of massage and aromatherapy in mental health appears to be: [the] alleviation of stress, particularly at times of crisis; providing a concrete experience of relaxation; aiding the counselling process and psychosocial development; providing an alternative source of pleasure or relaxation to people with substance dependence; [and] helping survivors of physical abuse to become comfortable with touch.
>
> Vickers (1996)

Functional problems and confusion

Many of our patients will experience confusion and this has been defined as:

> A temporary state of fluctuating intellectual impairment characterised (and recognised) by some or all of the following features – disorientation in time or space, impaired concentration and attention span, inability to register new memories and imperfect comprehension of surrounding events.
>
> Kendell (1988)

This is only an organic symptom or mild impairment of consciousness and is often termed a 'confusional state'. This implies a condition in which attention and thinking are impaired. But where more severe disturbance of consciousness and cognition, including difficulties with perception, it is suggestive of delirium. Such acute disturbances are caused by a variety of physical and psychological factors and determining the cause, apart from where there is a history of head injury or stroke, is extremely difficult. At one time most delirium was caused by infectious diseases, but now the cause tends to be drug or alcohol related.

Confusion is present in many clinical situations and it may be caused by cerebral ischaemia and hypoxia, metabolic disorders such as electrolyte imbalance, porphyria, hypoglycaemia, vitamin deficiency, endocrine disorders, head injury, epilepsy, space-occupying lesions, vascular emergencies, mental health problems, or any infections and toxicity. Clinical signs of confusion are therefore extremely varied within older people and may include any disruption of their routine, being introduced to unfamiliar environments, medical treatments, sensory deprivation, pain, pharmacotherapy, falls and enforced immobility (Saunders 1995)

It seems that nurses working in general settings are not always able to appreciate the intricacies of confusion and sometimes feel that they are not educationally equipped to manage such patients (Holden 1995). This is aggravated by the fact that they often find it difficult to differentiate between temporary and progressive states and also may not be able to distinguish dementia, depression and acute confusion or delirium (Jordan and Torrance 1995). This skill may be very important to possess because evidence suggests that in both medical and surgical elderly patients, confusion may be experienced by between 25% and 51% (Saunders 1995). Holden (1995) also noted that there was a higher incidence of postoperative confusion for older people than in any other age group. They are also seen to suffer 'interval' postoperative confusion, where they appear fully conscious after surgery and are able to respond normally but after a few days show signs of rambling. As this appears to be aggravated by the stresses associated with hospitalisation, such patients need to be carefully assessed and monitored, ideally by specialist nurses!

Organic illness

Alzheimer's disease is the most common and most well-known form of dementia. A report *Home Alone: Living with dementia* by the Alzheimer's Disease Society (ADS) (Keady 1994) highlighted that, of the estimated 636 000 people with dementia in the UK, 154 000 live alone and half of these will be over 85. The number living alone is, however, expected to rise to 245 000 by 2011. The report suggests that health authorities have failed adequately to identify and monitor individuals with dementia living alone, and that this has led to diminishing services for them and that they are subsequently a very vulnerable population. It also revealed that services to such patients seemed to concentrate on home helps and meals on wheels, and that 28% of those living alone received no professional visits. It has also been estimated that there are approximately 15 000 sufferers between the ages of 40 and 64 years (Cayton 1993).

Alzheimer's disease is characterised by diseased and/or dead brain nerve cells causing progressive mental function deterioration. Some research suggests that altered genes (changing one of the brain's proteins) may be responsible. Others suggest that aluminium affects this, or that extra β-amyloid (plaques) may be responsible. Early detection is problematic because forgetfulness and confusion may just be attributed to 'normal' ageing. Short-term memory loss is present in Alzheimer's disease and loss of reasoning and thinking becomes more marked. Such deterioration, which is individually influenced, is irreversible and leads to eventual death. As many of the symptoms such as nutritional deficiency and depression are common to other diseases, there is no true diagnostic technique. Although brain scans, and neuropsychological and neuro-physical tests all guide diagnosis, it often relies on the exclusion of other disorders and is only confirmed at *post mortem*.

As current treatment aims at reducing the consequences of this disease, complementary therapies may have some part to play in easing the anxiety, depression and sleep problems, and also the support of carers. It is very pertinent to consider the needs of such lay carers because it has been estimated by the ADS that, of the 6 million looking after such patients, more than half will be doing this for over 80 hours each week and because of this 97% of them are anticipated to have some emotional problems. This burden of caring appears to have been exacerbated by a demise in respite facilities, which in turn leads to the onus of care being left increasingly with these lay carers.

Treatment

You may find it useful to use the treatment advice on associated disorders, etc. in other chapters. As carers will also benefit from many of these approaches, please refer to the discussion of this in Chapter 14.

Mental health, emotional and neurological treatments

Rose (1998) suggested that aromatherapy is extremely helpful in alleviating some of the symptoms such as confusion, aggression and anger in patients suffering from not only Alzheimer's disease but also other mental health problems. She advocated that a selection of the following essential oils should be used either as a synergistic blend or as a 'simple', where only one oil is used at a time:

Cananga odorata (ylang ylang): to soothe anger and grief
Citrus bergamia (bergamot): for anxiety
Rosemarinus officinalis (rosemary): for apathy
Salvea sclarea (clary sage): for depression
Picea mariana (spruce): for lethargy
Pelargonium graveolens (geranium): for fear
Rosa spp. (rose): for low self-esteem
Cupressus sempervirens (cypress): for loss (death)
Citrus aurantium (neroli): for mental stress
Jasminum officinalis (jasmine): to stimulate.

She advocated that the essential oils were administered as an inhalation, via a compress, in a lotion, or in a massage blend. Mantle (1996), Brown (1993), Price and Price (1995), Worwood (1994) and Davis (1999) all noted that *Rosemarinus officinalis* was useful where there was loss of memory and other sensory deficits such as confusion and reduced concentration. Hudson (1996) also noted that there was some evidence to suggest that *Lavandula angustifolia* (lavender) had the same sedating effect as chlorpromazine but without leaving the patient feeling lethargic the following day. (See Chapter 12 for a case study, which shows some caution in the choice and use of essential oils when trying to help a patient with Alzheimer's disease to rest.)

Walsh and Wilson (1998) investigated the benefits of relaxation, aromatherapy, reflexology, and joint aromatherapy and reflexology sessions on their severely disabled, long-stay neurology patients. The researchers were keen to establish whether any of the therapies could positively influence pain, mood or perceived physical health in them. Treatments occurred once a week for 5 weeks. The order of treatment was randomised across participants and assessors were blind to the treatment. As the patients all had postural problems and suffered frequent spasms, it was impossible to treat them on a couch so they, except for two patients, received back massage. They were treated while sitting either in their wheelchairs or in their own beds.

Generally patients reported that they had received considerable benefits from each of the four treatments, but the highest daily mood ratings were recorded while they were within the combined aromatherapy and reflexology phase. The researchers concluded that overall there was some evidence to suggest that their patients could benefit from such approaches. The therapies continue and treatments are now formally evaluated.

Case study of a bereaved stroke patient

Tony, aged 75 years, suffered a right-sided stroke with a left hemiplegia and hemianopia. He was transferred to the stroke unit from his original hospital within 1 week. He progressed well and was discharged home into the care of his much younger sister. He had never married and had no other family. Six days after discharge his sister unfortunately died. The bereft patient was admitted to a nursing home for short-term care. As a result of his understandable depression, he attended a day hospital 3 days a week and restarted physiotherapy and occupational therapy. He was an extremely brave man but it was particularly difficult to discuss progress with him because he became upset and tearful very easily. He never mentioned his sister and decried the home in which he was staying. He longed to return home but was unable both mentally and physically to care for himself. He developed good relationships with the day hospital staff especially the occupational therapist (OT) and became very protective of other patients.

I saw this patient at the request of the care home team, because they were very anxious about his increasing withdrawal from the home's activities. As he was reluctant to have any physical contact with me, however, I thought it appropriate only to make a blend of oils for his personal use. I chose oils that would not only alleviate his physical pain but also help his spiritual and emotional pain. I chose a synergistic blend of *Citrus bergamia* because, although it has antidepressant properties, it is also uplifting, *Juniperus communis* (juniper), which acts as a cleanser for those with 'emotional stagnation' (Armstrong and Heidingsfeld 2000), and *Cupressus sempervirens*, which is useful for grief and also acceptance of change. These all had the added advantage of being male aftershave-type smells.

I also asked the home to purchase the Bach flower remedies walnut, to help him adapt to his changed circumstances, and honeysuckle because it helps those rooted in the past to 'move on.' He readily accepted the oil mix and applied it twice daily. He has been using this blend for 3 months now and the OT, who monitors him when she visits, has noticed some relaxation of his mood and a greater acceptance of his situation. Of course part of this could be to do with the passage of time since his sister died. (More is said in Chapter 11 about stroke patients.)

Multiple sclerosis

Patients with multiple sclerosis, a chronic disease of the central nervous system, seem to be increasingly seeking help for their symptoms from alternative and complementary therapies. One very small-scale American study sought to explore this (Fawcett et al. 1994). They found that the most frequent treatments accessed were nutritional, counselling, physical and massage therapies, and just under one-third of them reported that they had improved their quality of life. Interestingly, two-thirds of the respondents stated that they had chosen such treatments because orthodox practice could offer them no cure!

As Joyce and Richardson (1997) had built up a collection of case studies on the beneficial use of reflexology with their patients with multiple sclerosis, they sought to investigate whether a wider population could also benefit. The reflexology study group received 1 hour of reflexology for 12 weeks. Their symptoms were assessed, using a simple form of 19 categories, during their first treatment, and at 6 and 12 weeks to see if these symptoms had changed. The control group received no reflexology and their symptoms were assessed in the same way.

At 6 weeks, most of the reflexology group showed significant improvement in many of their symptoms and most of this was maintained at 12 weeks. Reflexology treatments then stopped and they were reassessed after a further 6 weeks; only very few of the patients had maintained this improvement. In fact some of them regressed to the level at the start of the study or even worsened. Although there were natural variations of symptomatology in the control group, there were no significant changes observed. The report concluded that there is some short-term benefit in regular reflexology, especially in relation to improvements in bladder control, sleep, circulation and relief of constipation.

Another small study (Graydon and McKee 1997) sought to examine whether massage therapy could offer multiple sclerosis patients any appreciable benefits. The patients each received a 25-minute back and leg oil massage given by qualified therapists and there was no control group. Mood states, including tension, depression, anger, fatigue and vigour, were tested pre- and post-intervention, immunological effects were monitored, and participants were also asked to record their own perceptions of treatment, using one-word answers. The results revealed not only significant positive changes in mood states but also that immune functioning could be noticeably improved. The researchers felt that the psychological and immune function improvements could also be of benefit to patients with non-multiple sclerosis conditions.

Special needs populations

Aromatherapy has been used with clients with impaired communication. Armstrong and Heidingsfeld (2000) were invited to provide aromatherapy for a mixed age group of profoundly disabled deaf and deaf–blind people, many of whom had not only sensory and cognitive losses but also physical disability. The aim of treatment was to aid relaxation, improve communication skills and general level of health, and provide them with 'a nice treat'. In addition to this, residents were encouraged to make choices about their own treatment. Perceived benefits appear, so far, to include a less fearful (especially about touch) and more relaxed empowered client group who have also begun to display some early signs of enhanced communication skills. It has also led to tremendous interest within the unit's staff and the scheme continues using a very specific and clear protocol for practice (refer to Chapter 1 for guidance).

Sanderson and Carter (1994) used aromatherapy and massage to introduce more expressive touch into the lives of their clients. These clients all had severe learning disabilities and touch was often the only means they had of communicating and self-expression. Essential oils were added so that the aromas could provide further sensory stimulation. Although they experienced some initial difficulties in massaging such clients and results were slow to achieve, the authors felt that the treatment had the potential to deepen trusting relationships among them all.

Relaxation was taught to patients with challenging behaviour at Rampton Hospital. Dangerous, violent or criminal patients are sent to Rampton where they are detained and divided into three directorates within which appropriate treatment is initiated, depending on their condition and need. Many of the patients had already followed behavioural modification programmes but were still displaying aggressive, agitated and disruptive behaviour, which both disturbed other residents and prevented any meaningful therapy being done.

The relaxation techniques chosen had to be uncomplicated and tailored to each resident's level of ability. It proved very challenging for them to teach relaxed postural positions because the patients tended to spend much of their time 'hunched up', rocking to and fro or in other defensive positions. The relaxation sessions were conducted in a quiet, specially equipped room. Initially many of the residents ran shouting around the room but after a while the sessions became quieter and new therapy approaches emerged. Of 15 patients who received sessions, all but two have progressed.

Sensory activities for older people with sensory loss

A colleague and I have tried to stimulate and trigger reactions from some older, mentally infirm residents of a nursing home. Our aim was to enhance their quality of life and create a healing environment of care, and to do this we have actively engaged them in the following multisensory activities:

1. Blending of aromatic lotions, bath gels, spritzers – these are formulated to their individual preference.
2. Memory and tactile stimulation with herbs, spices and essential oils and may include making articles such as scented sachet pillows – these activities encompass the feeling and smelling of various substances and can be both challenging and fun for the residents.
3. Experiencing scented touch via facials, footbaths, and hot scented flannels and towels – these activities can be very pleasurable for the residents but also have the power to evoke various reactions because of the power of touch and the evocative smells (see Chapter 2 for the role of touch and Chapter 4 for olfaction and smell).

Most of the residents appeared to benefit from these activities in several ways. They enjoyed participating in the activities because it provided them with not only mental and physical stimulation, but also gifts that they could share with their relatives and each other.

What are the implications of introducing such activities to vulnerable patients/clients?
How would you introduce sensory activities to your client/patient group?
What would encourage or deter you from doing this?

Emotional distress

A survey conducted by the Mental Health Foundation, looking at how people in emotional distress took control of their lives, included an analysis of alternative and complementary (CAM) therapy usage (Faulkner 1997). Their definition of CAM was very broad and originally included the 'talking therapies'. Eventually these were excluded because so many more clients had experienced these than other CAM therapies. The research revealed that most people surveyed had experience of talking, leisure, and art and creative therapies. When asked about the perceived benefits, increased relaxation and relief of stress and tension were identified as being of most benefit. The report also noted that many of these clients also felt that they were treated more as 'a whole person', and allowed to take more responsibility for their own health than within statutory mental health service provision. As a result of this, recommendations were made that funding should be made available so that clients are afforded the opportunity of accessing appropriate therapies that have been clearly negotiated.

Tension/stress/relaxation

A few studies have attempted to look at the alleviation of stress and anxiety. Van der Riet's (1993) study showed that massage reduced preoperative anxiety in a group of gynaecological patients who were between 18 and 85 years, and Ferrell-Tory and Glick (1993) found that massage helped alleviate pain and anxiety, even in terminally ill people.

Saeki (2000) investigated the effect of a foot soak, with or without lavender (genus not specified), on the autonomic nervous system (ANS). The results showed that, although there were no heart or respiratory changes, there was some significant increase in parasympathetic nerve activity for both types of footbath. With the addition of lavender, there was some relaxation in the ANS.

Groer et al. (1994) claimed that just a 10-minute nursing back massage could have a significant effect on patients' biochemical healing processes, both by alleviating anxiety and by stimulating the production of antibodies. Although the randomly selected samples of 18 participants and 14 control group patients were small, the researchers found that, although both groups had reduced anxiety levels post massage, the treatment group also had raised immunoglobulin in their saliva. Both studies concluded that it would therefore be worthwhile to incorporate massage therapy more fully into nursing practice.

Massage has also been shown to help reduce stress in the work place (Lewis 1995) and, although the research studied midwives, it may still be pertinent to consider for those working in other clinical areas. The results revealed that over half of the staff members who participated in the study felt that they were poorly supported at work and that they dealt with their problems by talking to others about them. After a 20-min massage all the participants' pulse rates dropped by an average of 12 beats/min and all felt more relaxed.

The normalising of emotions

Essential oils are very valuable to help normalise emotions and I have found the following very useful: *Lavandula angustifolia* is soothing, relaxing and calming; *Santalum album* helps relieve depression and anxiety; citrus oils such as *Citrus reticulata* (mandarin), *Citrus paradisi* (grapefruit) and *Citrus vulgaris* (orange) are calming, uplifting and refreshing; and *Rosa damascena* (rose) is particularly helpful for stress and shock. I have also found the following blends useful: *Boswellia thurifera* (frankincense), *Lavandula angustifolia* and *Santalum album* to aid relaxation; *Citrus bergamia*, *Citrus aurantifolia* (lime) and *Rosemarinus officinalis* to combat fatigue, and *Salvea sclarea*, *Citrus bergamia*, *Anthemis nobilis* (Roman chamomile) and *Santalum album* to ease stressful occasions. All of these may be used within massage therapy, added to the bath or diffused into the atmosphere. I feel that they are particularly useful made up into a cream or oil, and applied to tense areas of the body, such as the temples, or neck and shoulders.

Reflexology therapy could include a generalised 'balancing' treatment followed by massage to the specific and related reflex zones affected. Tanner (1990) advocates treating the solar plexus, pituitary gland, thyroid and parathyroid, lungs, kidney, spine, shoulder, hip, leg and the lymphatic reflexes to elicit stress reduction.

Bach flower remedies

These are particularly useful for releasing negative emotions and dealing with stressful situations. It would be impossible to mention them all here, because probably, at some time, all would be valuable to use. Instead, I would refer you to Chapter 6 where they are all listed. The choice will depend on the condition, needs and experiences of the individual patient (Howard 1990). The composite Rescue Remedy, olive, crab apple, aspen, hornbeam, vervain and walnut remedies are likely to be of use to many patients with emotional imbalance.

A disappointing encounter with a patient with chronic fatigue syndrome

This is added here to remind you that not all encounters with patients are successful! Sylvia, aged 61, had been a very successful pianist but, because she had started experiencing severe tiredness, 'anxiety' and coordination problems, she was forced to retire prematurely and against her wishes. She was extremely angry about this, but she kept her emotions well hidden. She had consulted several 'specialists' to no avail and as a last resort came to see me.

For her treatment I used *Citrus aurantium* for her anxiety, *Jasminum officinale* because it is useful for those with psychological and psychosomatic disorders and also lethargy and sadness, *Lavandula angustifolia* (lavender) for its analgesic properties, and *Anthemis nobilis* for its anti-inflammatory, balancing and calming properties.

She was given a complete massage treatment. Her shoulders were initially stiff and tender, but she had no stiffness in her neck or other joints. She went to sleep at the start of treatment and remained asleep afterwards. She seemed extremely relaxed and was much more mobile than when she had arrived. After treatment I gave her the same oils to take home and advised her to drink plenty of water and not to engage in any heavy lifting.

She rang the next day to say that her treatment had been 'a waste of time'. I understand that she is still seeking an answer elsewhere for her problems.

Headaches and migraine

Many people suffer from headaches and migraines and they can be very troublesome because they often have a tremendous impact on a person's quality of life. Although Pope (1997) estimated that over 4 million people in Britain suffered from migraine alone, Vernon et al. (1999) noted that current population-based studies had reported that tension-type headaches occurred in approximately 35–40% of the adult Western population! As a consequence of this, they reviewed the randomised controlled trials (RCTs) of CAM therapies in the treatment of non-migrainous type headaches (i.e. they excluded cluster, migraine and organic headaches). They found that most of the studies had involved acupuncture and concluded that, as some of these RCTs were rigorously conducted, there appeared to be limited evidence that some CAM therapies could be useful in the treatment of the most common forms of headache.

Although the study of Puustjarvi et al. (1990) suggested that back massage could alleviate migraine, it seems that reflexology may also have a role to play in the relief of headaches. One Danish study (Brendstrup et al. 1996) investigated the potential of reflexology to help with the relief of migraine and tension-type headaches. The study excluded people with serious illness and involved 220 participants and 78 reflexologists from all over Denmark; 90% had been on medication for their headaches within 1 month of the start of the study. After a course of treatment 23% of the participants reported that they were symptom free and 55% of them stated that both the severity and the frequency of their symptoms were reduced. At follow-up 3 months later only 10% revealed that they had been completely cured, although 68% felt that their symptoms were far less severe and 19% had been able to stop their analgesia.

Case study of a patient with a complex history of symptoms, including headache

Charlie is a 65-year-old retired teacher who now leads a very sedentary yet stressful life. Her diet is very erratic and poor, but she smokes and drinks only socially. She has two adult children both born in the 1950s and an inconsequential past medical history, but has recently been diagnosed with a hiatus hernia. She takes antacids, as required for dyspepsia, and laxatives daily for constipation. She is also overweight, with a body mass index (BMI) of 31, which she claims is a result of taking long-term migraine medication (Sanomigran). She has cluster-type headaches almost daily. She has some residual cold symptoms and her sinuses appear to be blocked.

Initial visit

This obese tired woman was still suffering the after-effects of a cold, but was seeking help for generalised tiredness, chronic migraine and constipation, and also for her failure to lose weight while on her current medication for constipation. As she was evidently very toxic I chose to use 1 drop of *Juniperus communis* per 10 ml of composite carrier oil to initiate the cleansing process, but also to re-energise her both physically and emotionally. To this I added 1 drop of *Foeniculum vulgare* (fennel) to aid toxic elimination further, but also to address her problems of indigestion and constipation. Finally this was combined with 1 drop of *Melaleuca leucadendron* (cajuput) to clear her sinuses. Charlie was massaged, paying careful attention to the lower and upper lymphatics, sinus areas of the face and also her abdomen. Clockwise firm effleurage was applied here. The corresponding reflex zones were treated on her feet. After treatment she coughed a lot and her eyes and nose ran. She was advised to drink plenty of water and to continue with 2 drops of cajuput in a steam inhalation for her residual sinusitis. For her headaches, she was also given a mix of *Lavandula angustifolia*, *Mentha piperita* (peppermint) and *Salvea sclarea*, 2 drops of each in 30 ml of carrier oil, and advised to massage this into her temples. She agreed to return in 2 weeks.

Second visit

Charlie returned and stated that her sinusitis had improved but was very disappointed that her constipation was no better. I explained that, as she had suffered this problem for a long time, it might take several treatments before any results were noted. I substituted 1 drop of *Pogostemon patchouli*

(patchouli) for the *Melaleuca leucadendron*, because it is very useful for an atonal bowel. I omitted the sinus area on both the face and feet, and continued as before, adding extra pressure massage to the cellulite on the outer thigh. After treatment she was advised again to drink plenty of fluid and also to increase the fruit and vegetables in her diet to aid bowel evacuation She took the remainder of the oil home for her bath and continued with the 'headache blend'. She would return in 2 weeks.

Third visit

As she was still feeling tired I gave her a mixture of two Bach flower remedies: olive for exhaustion and crab apple for self-disgust, because I could see that she felt very ashamed of her body. I continued as before but added 1 drop of the feminine *Rosa damascena* to lift her spirits. After treatment she said she felt less miserable and more relaxed and asked to come in 1 week. She was to continue the dietary measures and use the 'headache mix' as previously advised.

Fourth visit

Charlie was very pleased because she had managed to lose two pounds in weight, but her bowels were still very troublesome. I continued the therapy and oils as before but substituted the *Foeniculum vulgare* with 1 drop of *Origanum marjorana* (marjoram) because together they can act as a powerful laxative, especially if emotions play a part in such constipation. *Origanum marjorana* could also help her headaches. She chose to try this mixture of oils as an abdominal rub and would return in 3 weeks.

Fifth visit

Charlie had again lost a little weight and had a bowel action without taking her laxatives. She was anxious to continue as before and also to take the same mixture home to act as an abdominal rub; her headaches, she noticed, had also been less frequent. I advised her not to stop taking her medication without consulting her GP. She would continue her dietary regimen and return in 2 weeks.

Sixth visit

Charlie had progressed as for the fifth visit and was keen to keep the treatment regimen the same. After treatment Charlie felt less bloated than before and stressed that she would continue her dietary regimen and abdominal rub as before. She is especially pleased that her headaches have virtually disappeared, but was given a bottle of the 'headache mix' as a standby to apply at the first hint of a headache.

She continues to treat herself at home (hopefully)!

To conclude

This chapter has managed to address only a few of the complexities associated with the vast amount of conditions that have the potential to be helped by complementary approaches. Undoubtedly some of the problems highlighted are far reaching and all embracing for both patient and carer alike, but as Mantle (1996) said:

> If some of the barriers to communication can be reduced by [the] use of complementary therapies, nurses need to seize the opportunity to incorporate these into clinical practice.
>
> Mantle (1996)

References

Armstrong F, Heidingsfeld V (2000) Aromatherapy for deaf and deaf-blind people living in residential accommodation. Complementary Therapies in Nursing and Midwifery 6: 180–188.

Bond M (1988), cited in Kendell & Zealley (1988).

Brendstrup E, Launso L, Erikson L (1996) Denmark researches into headaches. Reflexions 42: 10.

Brown D (1993) Headway Guides: Aromatherapy. London: Hodder & Stoughton .

Cayton H (1993) Alzheimer's: ageing painfully. Practice Nurse 1–13 July, 291–293.

Davis P (1999) Aromatherapy an A–Z, revised edn. Saffron Walden: CW Daniel Co. Ltd.

Deakin M (1995) Using relaxation techniques to manage disruptive behaviour. Nursing Times 91(17): 40–41.

Faulkner A (1997) Knowing Our Own Minds. A survey of how people in emotional distress take control of their own lives. London: The Mental Health Foundation.

Fawcett J, Sidney J, Hanson M, Riley-Lawless K (1994) Use of alternative health therapies by people with multiple sclerosis: an exploratory study. Holistic Nursing Practice 8(2): 36–42 .

Ferrell-Tory A, Glick O (1993) The use of therapeutic massage as a nursing intervention to modify anxiety and the perception of cancer pain. Cancer Nursing 16: 93–101.

Graydon J, McKee N (1997) Massage as therapy in multiple sclerosis. International Journal of Alternative and Complementary Medicine 15(7): 27–28.

Groer M, Mozingo J, Droppleman P et al. (1994) Measures of salivary secretory immunoglobulin A and state anxiety after a nursing back rub. Applied Nursing Research 7(1): 2–6.

Holden U (1995) Dementia in acute units: confusion. Nursing Standard 9(17): 37–39.

Howard J (1990) The Bach Flower Remedies Step by Step. Saffron Walden: CW Daniel Co. Ltd.

Hudson R (1996) The value of lavender for rest and activity in the elderly patient. Complementary Therapies in Medicine 4: 52–57.

Jordan S, Torrance C (1995) Bionursing: confusion in elderly people. Nursing Standard 10(6): 30–32.

Joyce M, Richardson R (1997) Reflexology can help MS. International Journal of Alternative and Complementary Medicine 15(7): 10–12.

Keady J (1994) Living alone with dementia. British Journal of Nursing 3: 648–9.
Kendell R (1988), cited in Kendell and Zealley (1988).
Kendell R, Zealley A (1988) Companion to Psychiatric Studies, 4th edn. Edinburgh: Churchill Livingstone.
Lewis L (1995) Caring for carers. Modern Midwife 5(2): 7–10.
McGregor I, Bell J (1993) Voyage of discovery. Nursing Times 89(36): 29–31.
Mangan P (1996) Age Concern. Nursing Times 92(2): 47.
Mantle F (1996) Contact points. Nursing Times 92(18): 46–47.
Norman I (1992) Depression in old age. In: Redfern S, ed., Nursing Elderly People, 2nd edn. Edinburgh: Churchill Livingstone.
Pope N (1997) Yes, tonight dear … I've got a headache. RX7 September.
Price S, Price L (1995) Aromatherapy for Health Professionals. Edinburgh: Churchill Livingstone.
Puustjarvi K, Airaksinen O, Pontinen P (1990) The effects of massage in patients with chronic tension headaches. Acupuncture Electrotherapy Research 15: 159–162.
Rose J (1998) Alzheimer's disease: An aromatherapy overview. Aromatherapy Quarterly 56: 33–35.
Saeki Y (2000) The effect of footbath with or without the essential oil of lavender on the autonomic nervous system: a randomized trial. Complementary Therapies in Nursing and Midwifery 8: 2–7.
Sanderson H, Carter A (1994) Healing hands. Nursing Times 90(11): 46–48.
Saunders P (1995) Caring for confused people in the general hospital setting. Nursing Times 91(47): 27–29.
Tanner R (1990) Step by Step Reflexology. Surrey: Douglas Barry.
Van der Riet (1993) Effects of therapeutic massage on pre-operative anxiety in a rural hospital – part 1. Australian Journal of Rural Health 1(4): 11–16.
Vernon H, McDermaid C, Hagino C (1999) Systematic review of randomized clinical trials of complementary/alternative therapies in the treatment of tension-type and cervicogenic headache. Complementary Therapies in Medicine 7: 144–155.
Vickers A (1996) Massage and Aromatherapy: A guide for health care professionals. London: Chapman & Hall.
Walsh E, Wilson C (1998) Complementary therapies in long-stay neurology in-patient settings. Nursing Standard 13(32): 32–35.
Worwood V (1994) The Fragrant Pharmacy. London: Bantam Books.

Further reading

Brown D (1993b) Headway Guides: Massage. London: Hodder & Stoughton.
Price S, Price L (1995) Aromatherapy for Health Professionals. Edinburgh: Churchill Livingstone.
Snyder M, Egan E, Burns K (1995) Efficacy of hand massage in decreasing agitation behaviors associated with rare activities in people with dementia. Geriatric Nursing March/April: 60–63.
Snyder M, Egan E, Burns K (1995) Interventions for decreasing agitation behaviors in persons with dementia. Journal of Gerontological Nursing July: 35–40.

CHAPTER 8
Respiratory and circulatory conditions

By working together, the respiratory and cardiovascular systems ensure an adequate supply of oxygen to the tissues and the removal of carbon dioxide from the body. The cardiovascular system is also responsible for transporting substances such as hormones, nutrients and waste products around the body. During ageing several structural changes, which affect effective functioning, occur in the chest and lungs.

As one ages there is a loss of respiratory function, which is substantially greater in people who smoke than in those who don't. As some return in function is possible if smokers give up, it seems sensible to encourage this in older people when respiratory function is already compromised. In the lung, there is a reduction in both the lung volume and capacity with a correspondingly reduced surface area available for gaseous exchange and, because of stiffening of the collagen, there is some loss of elasticity. As a result of this and other regressive structural changes within the thorax, more muscular work is needed to move air in and out of the lungs. Respiratory defence mechanisms are also less effective. The cilia or the fine hair-like projections on the bronchial epithelium are reduced and the motility of those remaining is less powerful, so mucus and foreign bodies are less readily expelled. This accounts partly for the increase in respiratory infections in elderly people. Complementary therapies may be able to respond to and alleviate many of the above changes identified in the respiratory tract.

General principles of treatment

Colds, coughs, catarrh, influenza, rhinitis and sinusitis will all benefit from reflexology because it often causes an increase in excretory action, and may therefore act as a very efficient decongestant. Treatment will include a cursory exploration of all the reflex points, followed by an in-depth treatment of respiratory, skeletal, circulatory and excretory systems (see Chapter 5 for the full procedure). The inhalation of essential oils is also very effective for these conditions and, as the dosage and methods of application have been well covered in Chapter 3, only the specifics of treatment are presented below.

Colds, coughs, catarrh, sinusitis, rhinitis and influenza

As we know full well, there is no cure for the common cold, so the measures adopted for treatment merely act to relieve the symptoms and try to prevent secondary infection. The essential oils of *Styrax benzoin* (benzoin), *Melaleuca leucadendron* (cajuput), *Eucalyptus globulus* (eucalyptus), *Lavandula angustifolia* (lavender), *Mentha piperita* (peppermint) and *Rosemarinus officinalis* (rosemary) are all suitable, even when bronchial catarrh and congestion are present. If the catarrh is caused by pollen and other allergens, as for instance in hayfever, then *Lavandula angustifolia* and *Anthemis nobilis* (Roman chamomile) should be the preferred oils. Where patients are experiencing sinusitis, they would benefit from the above oils but because of the pain an oil with analgesic properties, such as *Mentha piperita*, must always be included in the blend. Patients with influenza may require a more prolonged treatment, but care should be taken not to overstimulate them in the acute stage of the illness. A warm bath with *Anthemis nobilis* and *Lavandula angustifolia* may both soothe their aches and pains and help them to sleep.

These oils are all ideally administered by steam inhalation, which may need to be administered five or six times a day to bring relief, but they are also effective when added to a bath. Essential oils such as *Melaleuca leucadendron* and *Mentha piperita* when combined in a carrier oil make an excellent and soothing rub, which if applied under the nose greatly aids breathing. Coughs respond particularly well to steam treatment with any of the above oils, but appear to be soothed best by *Styrax benzoin* and *Boswellia thurifera* (frankincense). Warm herbal teas with honey will also soothe any irritation in the throat. Where patients keep getting coughs and colds, it may be useful to add *Melaleuca alternifolia* (tea tree) to their treatments because it acts as an immune booster.

Herpes (cold sores)

Herpes are caused by a virus and tend to be both painful and unsightly. They are best treated by oils such as *Lavandula angustifolia* and *Melaleuca alternifolia*. Although it is considered unsafe to use essential oils undiluted, one drop dabbed on the lesion, several times over the course of a day, seems to hasten the healing process.

Case study

The following case study shows both the multiple pathologies of old age and the versatility of the essential oils. This allows for quite a few problems to be treated by a blend of very few essential oils.

William is an 80-year-old retired architect, with a past history of serious chest disease and bleeding duodenal ulcer many years ago. Currently he says his nose is constantly bunged up and he has some difficulty in breathing. At night he sleeps for approximately 7 hours, with three pillows, because of this, but still snores. He suffers from allergic rhinitis in summer with residual catarrh in winter. He eats a well-balanced diet and has a healthy appetite and opens his bowels twice daily. He has no problems with micturition and gets up once during the night to void urine. He suffers from a painful left knee and hip, but is unable to take anti-inflammatory drugs because of his predisposition to gastric bleeding. Difficulties occur particularly when he bends or tries to stand up from sitting. His skin is very sensitive and he is careful about what he puts on it. He has no known allergies and is on Tylex, which contains codeine and paracetamol, one to two tablets as required for pain.

Initial visit

This apparently very fit man presented with arthritic-type pain in his left knee and hip. He was most conscious that this slowed him down and prevented him from being as active as he would like to be. He was also irritated by his chronic sinusitis and resultant catarrh, especially as the associated constant nose blowing interfered with his eating. In an attempt to try to counteract all the apparent excess moisture in his body I added 1 drop of *Zingiber officinalis* (ginger) to 10 ml of composite base oil because this also has analgesic and anti-inflammatory properties, which would be beneficial for his arthritic pain and immobility. Then I added 1 drop of *Citrus limonum* (lemon) to disperse some of his acidity and toxicity. Finally 1 drop of *Styrax benzoin* (benzoin) was combined with the other two oils because of its mucus-expelling properties and special affinity with breathless elderly people. As he has a very sensitive skin, I was extra careful to mix in the lemon.

A generalised massage was given, paying particular attention to the knees and hips, lymphatic drainage, and the sinus and nasal areas of the face. The corresponding reflex zones were treated on both feet. After treatment William appeared very relaxed and his nose streamed with excess mucus. It was difficult to assess any improvement in his mobility. He was advised to have regular inhalations containing up to 4 drops of *Styrax benzoin* and to return in 1 week.

Second visit

William returned 8 days later clearly quite poorly with a streaming cold. He was still prepared to have treatment but, as he was evidently so full of infection, I massaged him very gently, substituting the *Citrus limonum* with *Melaleuca alternifolia* (tea tree). This I felt would cut down on the detoxification and help clear his residual infection. As he was so 'bunged up' he was propped up with several pillows. I massaged only the front of his limbs, both knee and hip joints, and sinus and nasal areas on his face. No reflexology was performed in case I overstimulated him. After treatment he coughed and produced copious mucus from his nose. He was advised to continue the inhalations of *Styrax benzoin* (2 drops) and *Melaleuca alternifolia* (2 drops) and to return when his infection had abated.

Third visit

Two weeks later he returned and said, although his cold was much better, he felt very cold and almost exhausted. I continued with the *Styrax benzoin* and *Zingiber officinalis*, omitted the *Melaleuca alternifolia* and added 1 drop of *Piper nigrum* (black pepper) for increased warmth. In addition I gave him 4 drops of the Bach flower remedy olive for his exhaustion and used the massage routine employed on his second visit. After treatment he stated that he felt much warmer and almost euphoric. His mobility appeared to be marginally improved and he said that, although his hip and knee felt stiff, they were pain free. I suggested that he might like to try some oils in his bath, but he said that he had not managed this in over 20 years and was too afraid to try now. I advised him to buy some olive and take regularly and also to continue with the *Styrax benzoin* inhalations if required, and to return in 2 weeks.

Fourth visit

He said that his mobility was much improved and thought that was because he had remained pain free for over a week. He was keen that I continue the treatment as of his second visit. In addition I mobilised his knee joints but omitted the olive because he was still taking his. After treatment he was pleased with the greater flexibility of his knees and, as he was feeling less fraught, said that he would continue with the olive for one more week and then tailor it off. He would also continue with the inhalations. He requested to return in 1 week, because he was afraid that the benefits he was experiencing would wear off.

Fifth visit

His improved mobility was quite marked and he was proud to show that he could bend again. His treatment continued as of the last visit. After treatment he requested whether the oils used could be put in a cream so that he could apply the warming mixture before retiring for the night, because it was then that his joints really ached. He would continue with this. I was concerned that he would overdose, because of his age, and suggested that he did not use both the cream and the inhalations simultaneously. He agreed to this. I suggested that he should return in 2 weeks.

> Evaluate the care given to the above patient and consider whether his problems were appropriately addressed.
> Could other measures have been used to make his treatment more effective?

His mobility was markedly improved, as was his sinus condition. Although he still needed to blow his nose a lot, the mucus was clear and not viscid and did not interfere so much with his eating. He felt very well after treatment and continues to be treated fortnightly.

Asthma

Asthma is a very common illness, which can be triggered by a host of different conditions, and involves long-term inflammation or swelling of the respiratory tract and is said to affect approximately 3.4 million people in the UK (National Asthma Campaign 2000). Yet a recent survey (Dow et al. 2001) found that one in five sufferers over the age of 65 might not be receiving any treatment for it. Although asthma is not a minor respiratory condition and still remains one of the major causes of hospital admission today, evidence suggests that patients do not like and therefore do not adhere to traditional treatments (Coakley 1999). I felt that it was useful to discuss here, because there are limited signs that such patients are seeking alternative treatments.

The National Asthma Campaign (1997) surveyed 4000 people with asthma and found that almost half (48%) of them had experimented with complementary therapies, but only a third of those said that they had improved their condition. On the basis of this, the National Asthma Campaign have recognised that some patients want to try other options and have tried to adopt a more integrated approach to care. They urge caution in this and warn that patients should not disregard orthodox medical advice because asthma still accounts for four deaths a day.

Vickers and Smith (1997) were, however, concerned about the lack of information readily available to inform practice about the effectiveness of complementary therapy treatments for asthma. In their conservative review of 35 papers, they found that most of them concerned acupuncture or self-regulation techniques and were small scale, and that treatments were often different to those used in everyday practice and mostly assessed only standard lung function.

Lewith (1996) suggests that, because asthma is a long-term problem and is on the increase, it would be sensible to encourage patients to adopt more self-treatment strategies, alongside orthodox approaches, both to limit and to improve the effects of their condition. He recommends the appropriate use of dietary management and mind–body therapies because they are potentially cost-effective methods of disease management. Rector-Page (1996) also advocates that patients devise an effective self-care programme, alongside their prescribed care, because she says that there is evidence to suggest that, by doing so, they may be able to limit their drug dependence. Such a programme would include: a mucus-cleansing liquid diet, herbal remedies to encourage antihistamine production, antioxidant supplementation and some type of bodywork therapy.

Any reflexology treatment will include contacting the upper skeletal points to relax the chest muscles, the respiratory points to aid breathing, and the circulatory, lymphatic and urinary reflexes to aid toxin removal. Ingham (1991) states that, as adrenaline is given for asthma in emergency situations, it is essential that these reflexes are stimulated. If essential oils are used, they should be chosen to treat both the physical and the underlying emotional manifestations of the disease. Such oils would ideally include: *Citrus bergamia* (bergamot), *Anthemis nobilis*, *Salvea sclarea* (clary sage), *Lavandula angustifolia*, *Rosa damascena* (rose) and *Citrus aurantium* (neroli) because they all have both antispasmodic and antidepressant properties. Bach flower remedies such as aspen, olive and holly may be useful to dispel any negative feelings.

Cardiovascular conditions

Normal ageing of the cardiovascular system varies substantially from individual to individual, but appears to be dependent on the amount of physical activity normally undertaken. There is a decline in the maximum heart rate that can be achieved with age but, despite some loss of cells in the sinoatrial node of the heart, the pacemaker function is not impaired. Blood flow to the kidneys and brain is reduced and there are also changes in resting blood flow to the myocardium and skeletal muscle. Although the changes affecting the latter two are less marked, the ability to increase blood flow to these tissues in an emergency is reduced in older people. As a result of changes within the capillary structure and an increased density of connective tissues, diffusion of gases and nutrients to and from the cells is impaired.

Blood pressure

There are marked changes in blood vessels during ageing. There is increased arterial stiffness and there is a loss of elasticity within the walls of the veins. This causes them to be weaker and may lead to varicosities if subjected to high pressure. There is also often an increase in systolic pressure with age, with a smaller increase in diastolic pressure. There is discussion about whether these increases are inevitably part of normal healthy ageing or a consequence of other dietary and social stresses. Diastolic pressure may fall in very old people.

Frankel (1997) studied the effect of reflexology on barocepter reflex sensitivity (BRS), blood pressure and sinus arrhythmia in a small population. One group (n = 10) received reflexology; another group (n =10) received foot massage and the control group (n = 4) had no therapeutic intervention at all. The results showed that both reflexology and foot massage reduced BRS substantially more than in the control group. As there was no mean difference between the two interventions, Frankel (1997) concluded that they may have a similar mechanical action. Although more subjective, the results did seem to suggest that both interventions caused an increase in sinus arrhythmia. As a result of discrepancies in the recording of the blood pressures, the results were deemed unsatisfactory.

Hypertension and hypotension

Essential oils are capable of both raising and lowering blood pressure. Suitable oils for the management of hypotension include: *Thymus vulgaris* (thyme) and *Rosemarinus officinalis* (rosemary). Two oils that may also help, but should be used less frequently are *Mentha piperita* and *Piper nigrum*, particularly where fainting is one of the problems (Davis 1999). These oils may be included in the massage blend.

Hypertensive episodes may be treated with *Lavandula angustifolia*, *Origanum marjorana* (marjoram) and *Cananga odorata* (ylang ylang). Davis (1999) notes that the last oil is particularly useful if there are associated breathing problems. Careful patient assessment is required before treating the above patients, because it is essential that you do not confuse the two conditions and select an inappropriate oil.

Stormer (1995) uses the following reflexology procedure on patients with hypertension. After a general treatment he concentrates on the whole of the central nervous system, and the endocrine, circulatory, respiratory, skeletal, lymphatic and urinary reflexes because the aim is to improve circulation and hasten toxin elimination from the body.

Varicose veins (see Chapter 9 for haemorrhoids)

This is a very painful condition, which often starts early in life and is found most commonly in women. Although many books advocate that massage should be avoided, because it may further damage the fragile capillary wall (Worwood 1994), Brown (1993) advises that patients may benefit enormously from the 'gentle and careful stroking' often used in aromatherapy massage. There may be some logic in this because the occurrence of varicose veins is very much influenced by poor circulation. Davis (1999) argues, however, that massage may be used only above the affected area and never below, because this will just increase the pressure in the vein.

Treatment should aim to improve circulation and there are several essential oils that are suitable for application. If I am concerned about using 'massage', I add the oils to warm water and apply as a compress instead. This is very soothing but also helps the itching, which so often accompanies this condition. Oils include: *Cupressus sempervirens* (cypress) for its astringency; *Mentha piperita* because it is cooling, analgesic and anti-inflammatory; and *Pelargonium graveolens* (geranium) for its bactericidal and anticoagulant properties.

I have looked only at the few cardiorespiratory conditions that I feel may be treated safely and competently with complementary therapies. Caution must be exercised within these systems because of the possible influence of allergic response and the presence of life-threatening illness. Minor problems can, however, be effectively relieved or eliminated, especially by the skilled use of essential oils and reflexology.

References

Brown D (1993) Headway Guides: Massage. London: Hodder & Stoughton.

Brown M (1994) The use of massage in restoring cardiac rhythm. Nursing Times 90(38): 36–37.

Coakley L (1999) Health Education and Asthma. Nursing Times Clinical Monograph 10. London: NT Books, Emap Healthcare Ltd.

Davis P (1999) Aromatherapy an A–Z, revised edn. Saffron Walden: CW Daniel Co. Ltd.

Dow L et al. (2001) Prevalence of untreated asthma in a population sample of 6000 older adults in Bristol. Thorax 15: 472–476.

Frankel B (1997) The effect of reflexology on the baroreceptor reflex sensitivity, blood pressure and sinus arrhythmia. Complementary Therapies in Medicine 5: 80–84.

Ingham E (1991) The Original Works of Eunice D. Ingham. Stories the feet can tell thru reflexology – Stories the feet have told thru reflexology (with revisions by Dwight C Byers). St Petersburg, FL: Ingham Publishing, Inc.

Lewith G (1996) Asthma: a complementary medical perspective. Complementary Therapies in Medicine 4: 106–111.

National Asthma Campaign (1997) Members' Survey. London: NAC.

National Asthma Campaign (2000). The National Asthma Campaign Audit Survey. London: NAC.

Price S, Price L (1995) Aromatherapy for Health Professionals. Edinburgh: Churchill Livingstone.

Rector-Page L (1996) Controlling Allergies and Overcoming Asthma with Herbs. New York: Healthy Healing Publications.

Stormer C (1995) Reflexology. The definitive guide. Reading: Hodder & Stoughton.

Tanner R (1990) Step by Step Reflexology. Surrey: Douglas Barry.

Vickers A, Smith C (1997) Analysis of the evidence profile of the effectiveness of complementary therapies in asthma: a qualitative survey and systematic review. Complementary Therapies in Medicine 5: 202–209.

Worwood V (1994) The Fragrant Pharmacy. London: Bantam Books.

Further reading

Beeken J, Parks D, Cory J, Montopoli G (1998) The effectiveness of neuromuscular release massage therapy in five individuals with chronic obstructive lung disease. Clinical Nursing Research 7: 309–325.

Brewin A (1998) Allergy avoidance. Nursing Standard 12(32): 49–56.

Brown D (1993) Headway Guides: Aromatherapy. London: Hodder & Stoughton.

Dunn C, Sleep J, Collett D (1995) Sensing an improvement: an experimental study to evaluate the use of aromatherapy, massage and periods of rest in an intensive care unit. Journal of Advanced Nursing 21(1): 34–40.

Jevon P, Ewens B (2001) Assessment of a breathless patient. Nursing Standard 15(16): 48–53.

Lewis P, Nichols E, Mackey G et al. (1997) The effect of turning and backrub on mixed venous oxygen saturation in critically ill patients. American Journal of Critical Care 6: 132–140.

Mantle F (1996) Opening up new relief routes. Nursing Times 92(10): 46–48.

Stevensen C (1994) The psychophysiological effects of aromatherapy massage. Complementary Therapies in Medicine 2(1): 27–35.

CHAPTER 9
Alimentary disorders

There are very few specific diseases associated with the ageing gastrointestinal tract. Although there are many changes and a progressive decline throughout adult life in many of the physiological functions associated with the alimentary tract, because of the reserve capacity within the system the function of the older gut is not normally impaired. Yet older people do tend to suffer from many minor symptoms associated with this system. Some of this may be socially or diet induced. This chapter therefore looks at the available approaches that may help to prevent or treat the most common symptoms of indigestion, flatulence, constipation and haemorrhoids, all of which must be thoroughly investigated before treatment to exclude serious pathology. It also considers loss of appetite, nausea and vomiting and the potential overuse of laxatives.

There are myths associated with the dietary needs of older people. Although it is true to say that both their food intake and their energy requirements diminish with increasing age, their nutrient requirements are similar to and in some instances even more than those of younger populations (Thomas 1992). As they tend to eat less, however, some of the essential nutrients are often missing from their diet. Further problems also arise because of either their inability or their reluctance to drink sufficient fluid (Nazarko 2000). As a direct consequence of both of these, nutritional deficiencies are frequently found in older patients.

As the precise recommended dietary allowances are not known for elderly people, it is sometimes difficult to establish how best to help them. Vitamin supplementation is often used to attempt to correct any deficiencies, improve the patient's appetite and also to promote a feeling of security. Nutritional deficiencies can be exacerbated by a whole range of events such as living alone, lack of interest in or need for food, poverty, the presence of confusion, simply because they are either edentulous or wearing ill-fitting dentures or the overuse of prescribed drugs. Drugs clearly impact on this system because of reduced metabolic and excretory efficiency. As a result of this, drugs tend to over-concentrate in the blood and a cumulative effect occurs. This is especially true of sedatives, opioids and opiate analgesics. Smaller doses are therefore required, especially because drug non-compliance and medication error are said to be greater in the older population.

Although, on the one hand, the under-utilisation of food is clearly a problem, on the other, if patients continue to eat the same amount of food as when they were younger, obesity may develop instead. This is equally as undesirable as weight loss because of the extra burden that increased weight will exert on both the cardiovascular system and the weight-bearing joints. Unfortunately, the advice given by both doctors and nurses relating to this is often very poor, confused or misinformed.

Dietary treatments

These treatments are based on the belief that health is inextricably linked to what we eat and this belief appears to be the basis of many therapies and treatment. Orthodox dietary advice has centred on the idea of a balanced diet, which includes the correct amounts of proteins, carbohydrates, fats, vitamins and minerals. Recently there has been a greater emphasis on reducing sugar, salt and fat, and at the same time increasing unrefined carbohydrates within the diet. Liu et al. (2000) examined the relationship between diet and stroke in 75 521 women who completed three questionnaires over a period of 10 years. They found that a diet rich in whole grains reduced the risk of stroke and, even if one daily serving of refined carbohydrates was replaced with whole grains, it appeared that there were still significant benefits.

The World Health Organization (WHO) and the Health Education Authority, to encourage healthy daily eating and stop people indulging in unhealthy diets, have become involved in this. They both note that specific diseases, including many of the cancers, may be prevented by or respond to dietary change, especially in relation to an increased daily allowance of fruit and vegetables (Wasling 1999). Yet Smith-Warner's (2001) recent large study did not support this because it found that fruit and vegetable consumption did not significantly reduce the risk of breast cancer.

Over the years, research has been sponsored to look at the role of diet in multiple sclerosis and as yet no proven factor has been isolated that irrefutably alters the course of this disease (Werbach 1997), although there is some evidence that the consumption of a low saturated fat diet might not only reduce the risk of developing the disease but have a positive influence on its progression. Similar fat-regulated diets have also shown limited benefits for patients with rheumatoid arthritis, not because diets low in saturated fat improve it, but because saturated fats aggravate the condition.

Complementary approaches to diet

Complementary advice is often incorporated into many therapies, but it is often contradictory and not in agreement with our past knowledge. Many of the therapists who offer such advice need not have had any formal training. Many also use 'risky practices' and claim that nutrition will cure all, e.g. one formal aromatherapy course I went on introduced us to various methods including a gallbladder-cleansing diet!

Gallbladder cleanse

Over a period of 24 hours the client is instructed to drink one-third of a pint of olive oil followed by the juice of one lemon, three times. After this the client is given a coffee enema to rid the body of green gallstones and so help detoxify the liver!

Many of these nutritional therapies tend to begin with fasting and cleansing measures such as colonic irrigation. Yet dietary advice has been given since very early civilisations, e.g. Hippocrates relied on liver as a source of nourishment and the early Babylonians and Greeks used garlic. By the eighteenth century limes were used to combat scurvy in the Navy, and during the nineteenth century vitamins and minerals were identified and synthesised. Complementary or alternative therapists work on the same principle that health is related to what we eat. Foods that have been used historically as medicine include: garlic for tuberculosis (TB), worms, colds and libido; grapes as a detoxifier and for constipation; and cherries for detoxifying, and stimulating sluggish systems. Some also suggest that certain foodstuffs, such as bananas, oats, liver and lettuce, will help our emotional health problems.

There are many different dietary therapies and I introduce you to five different ones below.

Nutritional medicine

Treatment is based on correcting imbalances in the quality and quantity of food eaten, the efficiency of digestion, absorption and utilisation of foodstuffs, and the patient's biochemical individuality. All of this is identified from the patient's dietary history, and treatment often concentrates on excluding many foods from a person's diet and then reintroducing them one at a time until the trigger for their problems is found (Booth 1993). Ballard (1996) who had been very debilitated by Crohn's disease, polyarthritis and menstrual problems embarked on such a strict regimen and noted how, within a month of treatment, she stopped all medication, apart from vitamin and mineral supplementation, because many of her symptoms had disappeared, and she was able to return to work. The best thing she found about the diet was that it gave her back control of her life!

Nutritional therapy

This is very similar to the above therapy because it also aims to explore the relationship between dietary factors and health, and then manipulate them so that the patient may benefit from optimal nutritional health. They concentrate on the identification of food allergy and intolerance, environmental toxicity, food sensitivity and nutritional deficits. Once a diagnosis is made, they seek to re-educate patients about their eating habits, put them on a modified diet and give nutritional supplements where necessary.

Gerson therapy

This is a dietary treatment, named after its developer, and based on the theory that environmental pollution, especially in relation to the food that we eat, causes many of our health problems. It claims to be beneficial to sufferers of cancer and arthritis and involves toxin identification, detoxification by the use of coffee enemas, the consumption of vast quantities of raw juices and nutritional supplementation.

Mega-vitamin therapy

As its name suggests, this therapy involves taking vast quantities of vitamins because it is thought that people do not access sufficient vitamins from their daily food intake. Currently, it is seen as very fashionable to take supplements, but there has been some controversy surrounding this therapy because some think the rationale behind it is flawed (Booth 1993).

Trophology

Food combining for health, which is strongly linked with Taoism, is advocated by many in relation to aromatherapy (Reid 1994). Taoists are against the simplistic Western theory of a balanced diet, because they feel that eating lots of different foods together is inefficient and encourages putrefaction and fermentation. This is called trophology or the science of food combining (Reid 1994), and modern diets such as the Hay diet are based on this philosophy. Taoists believe the following:

1. The balance between yin (cool/cold and calming) and yang (hot/warm and stimulating) is established by harmonising the four energies (hot, warm, cool, cold) and five flavours (sweet [earth], bitter [fire], sour [wood], pungent [metal], salty [water]) of food. Hot and cold extremes are avoided and food and drink are consumed separately. They therefore balance their diets according to favourable combinations of energies and flavour, and avoid combinations that conflict.
2. Excess consumption of any one food energy must be avoided.
3. Wherever possible local and fresh produce should be obtained.
4. Foods should be eaten that have a 'natural' affinity for their weakest organ.
5. They should eat to strengthen their organs and enhance sexual potency and longevity.
6. They eat meat sparingly and barely cooked.
7. They eat all foods sparingly and believe it is better to be only 70–80% full.
8. They must chew food many times as Ghandi said 'Drink your food and chew your beverages'.

Digestion

The mouth

After the age of 50, salivary flow diminishes in the mouth and there are fewer active taste buds, both of which may cause a decrease in appetite and an impaired nutritional intake. Dental decay and gum recession may lead to inadequate dentition and problems with oral hygiene.

Simple measures can help oral problems. Mouth washes containing essential oils can be used both to clean and to heal the oral cavity. The common oils that I use are *Melaleuca alternifolia* (tea tree) and *Citrus limonum* (lemon) for inflammatory and ulcerative conditions and *Commiphora myrrha* (myrrh) if a fungal infection is present. I would generally use 2 drops in half a tumbler of warm water and instruct the patient to gargle but not swallow the mixture. A salve, carefully applied, can help sore and cracked lips (see Chapter 4 for how to make this).

The ageing gut

As we age the stomach loses its muscular strength and tone and takes longer to empty, there is usually some decrease in secretions and acidity, and some individuals may also develop intolerance to foods such as fats. Although there is no evidence to suggest that absorption of major nutrients, such as amino acids, is impaired in healthy individuals, the villi in the small intestine shorten and become thicker which significantly reduces the surface area for absorption. You will find that many of the therapy books advocate that digestive remedies should be administered internally, but, as the lining of the alimentary mucosa could so easily be damaged by essential oils, it is not wise (Davis 1999). It is also currently not allowed by the major aromatherapy professional organisations.

Anorexia and reduced appetite

Thomas (1992) noted that anorexia or loss of appetite in older people deserves investigation because it is an important sign that their physical or emotional well-being is compromised. Although complementary therapies alone are unlikely to remedy this condition, they may prove useful in helping to create a conducive eating environment. Although the essential oils *Citrus bergamia*, *Piper nigrum* (black pepper), *Foeniculum vulgare* and *Zingiber officinale* (ginger) are useful as appetite stimulants, others such as *Cananga odorata* (ylang ylang) and *Jasminum communis* could scent the atmosphere. As a result of its uplifting and euphoric properties, *Citrus paradisi* (pink grapefruit) is considered by many to be the optimal appetite stimulant. Bach flower remedies, such as heather, honeysuckle, olive, wild rose, elm and star of Bethlehem, may be useful where there is an emotional cause to this problem.

Indigestion (dyspepsia)

This can be brought on by a variety of physical and emotional reasons. If it persists it should be investigated. Often it occurs because of a hurried lifestyle and poor eating practices. It is responsive to gentle abdominal massage with essential oils such as *Anthemis nobilis*, *Mentha piperita* (peppermint), *Lavandula angustifolia* (lavender), and *Origanum marjorana* (marjoram). Some patients find it helpful to drink peppermint, rosemary or fennel tea. Some dietary advice may also be necessary.

Nausea and vomiting

These can be very troublesome and may occur for many different physical and psychological reasons. As a result of this, Tanner (1990) feels that nausea can be alleviated by contacting the following reflex points: solar plexus, brain, ear and balance points, the stomach and large and small intestines, and the adrenal glands. Nausea may also be helped by the essential oils such as *Anthemis nobilis* (Roman chamomile), *Mentha piperita*, *Rosemarinus officinale* (rosemary) or *Lavandula angustifolia* either applied as a warm or cold compress to the head or by direct inhalation. After vomiting has ceased a cool and cleansing mouth wash of *Citrus limonum* or *Mentha piperita* may refresh the patient.

Flatulence

Flatulence may be associated with organic disease or, more commonly, is a result of swallowing too much air when eating or making a lot of intestinal gas during digestion. Where patients feel bloated, they may benefit from gentle abdominal massage or a reflexology treatment, which concentrates on the digestive, circulatory and lymphatic reflexes. Suitable essential oils that could be added to the abdominal rub include *Mentha piperita*, *Coriandrum sativum* (coriander) and *Eletteria cardamonum* (cardamon) (Worwood 1994). Drinking peppermint herbal tea is also helpful.

Obesity

Although obesity tends not to be a major problem in old age it does affect some people. Although it arises mostly from poor dietary intake, it is often emotionally influenced. Patients often feel ashamed of their large bodies and need help either to accept themselves as they are or to try to lose weight. Complementary therapies are extremely useful at this time because they can facilitate both of these. One must recognise, however, that false claims are still made about herbal drinks with anti-obesity properties (Madden 2000)! An example is now given of one patient's attempt to lose weight.

Case study of a patient trying to lose weight

Julie is a 68-year-old, retired, rather overweight woman with a body mass index (BMI) of 28 (the upper limit of normal is 25). She has been treated with thyroxine for many years for an underactive thyroid and is allergic to aspirin and nickel (gold).

Assessment revealed that she wants to lose weight and detoxify, and has recently commenced a food-combining diet but has not lost any weight as yet. Although she has reduced the dairy products in her diet, she still feels sluggish. Her appetite is good but not excessive and her bowel function is normal. Her skin is clear but ruddy.

Initial visit

This woman has some knowledge of aromatherapy and essential oils, but was keen to be massaged by someone other than herself. She was not concerned about her shoulder pain but was keen to lose weight and detoxify. She was adamant that a combination of *Foeniculum vulgare* (fennel), *Juniperus communis* (juniper) and *Vetiveria zizanoides* (vetivert) was used. I agreed these were very suitable for her needs (all three are very cleansing, both physically and emotionally, and eliminating) but when she actually smelt the combination (I drop of each per 10 ml of composite carrier oil) she did not like it, because it was very heavy. I added 1 drop of *Mentha piperita*, which altered the smell considerably. I felt the peppermint would also aid her sluggish digestion and act as an analgesic for her painful shoulder. In addition I gave her the Bach flower remedies crab apple, to reduce her emotional negativity, and hornbeam, to help her cope with her diet. She received a full general massage with robust lymphatic drainage plus extra clockwise effleurage to her abdomen. The corresponding reflex zones in her feet were also stimulated. She had recently commenced a food-combining diet and I advised her to continue with this. She took the remaining oils home to bathe in and would return in 1 week.

Second visit

Julie returned and stated that when she got home she felt quite bloated, had had a massive, fetid bowel action and that over the next 2 days her shoulder pain was better. I further discussed the oils with her and decided to continue with *Foeniculum vulgare* and *Juniperus communis*, but to omit the *Mentha piperita* and *Vetiveria zizanoides*. We decided to try I drop of *Boswellia thurifera* (frankincense) to lift her mood and also to relieve her latent flatulence. I continued to massage as before but only very gently massaged her abdomen. I excluded this from the reflex zone therapy but stimulated the head region. After treatment she was relaxed but still experiencing some flatulence. She would revisit after 1 week, meanwhile continuing on her diet. I also suggested that she drank more water.

Third visit

She had continued to have large, fetid stools. On enquiring, it seemed as though they were full of mucus. I therefore substituted the *Juniperus communis* with 1 drop of *Styrax benzoin* (benzoin) because of its mucus-expelling property. It is also an uplifting oil so it could continue to support her improved mental state. I adopted the regimen of her initial visit to try to clear her gut. She continued with the post-treatment advice and made an appointment for 2 weeks.

Fourth visit

Her skin was now very spotty and it appeared that she needed to leave the detoxifying alone for a few sessions. I therefore changed all her oils to the uplifting *Citrus bergamia* (bergamot) for her skin, *Anthemis nobilis* to quieten things down and *Salvia sclarea* (clary sage) to help her continue with her dieting (1 drop of each per 10 ml of composite carrier oil). Instead of a robust massage I applied soothing strokes to her back, limbs and face. After treatment she was relaxed and vowed to continue her diet. She agreed to return in 2 weeks.

Fifth visit

Her skin was less spotty and red and she had managed to lose about 3 kg. Treatment continued as before. She was relaxed and had no flatulence. She was continuing on her diet and would return in 3 weeks.

Sixth visit

Her skin was clear and she was delighted to have lost another kilogram. Treatment continued as above. She was now feeling far less sluggish and decided that she could use the remedies and massage techniques to help her. She was discharged and stated that she would return if she became demotivated when treating herself.

Elimination

Constipation

The symptom constipation appears to be one of the biggest problems that health carers have to deal with in older populations, especially when you also look at the associated problem of laxative abuse. It is estimated that the NHS in England alone spends approximately £43 million each year on prescription laxatives, but Bush (2000) feels that the actual expenditure is likely to be much higher because many others are purchased without prescription.

Constipation often arises because there is reduced peristaltic action within the intestines as a result of decreased muscle tone; consequently there is more faecal stasis. As the incidence of diverticula is increased and the elasticity of the rectal wall is reduced, the urge to defaecate becomes weaker. The lack of a high roughage diet and adequate fluids may also contribute to this. Commonly, older people become obsessed with daily bowel activity and resort to taking over-the-counter preparatory laxatives; it seems that between 20% and 30% of people over the age of 65 are regular users (Bush 2000).

Dietary measures should be instigated wherever possible and the use of laxatives should be discouraged. Increasing bulking agents in the diet of older people is, however, often unsatisfactory because it does not always relieve their constipation, and may leave them with faecal incontinence and abdominal distension (Bush 2000). Where constipation continues to be unresolved, abdominal massage has been found to be useful. Several authors (Emly 1993, Resende et al. 1993, Emly et al. 1998) have investigated this. One study by Resende et al. (1993) found that abdominal massage not only increased daily bowel motions, but also reduced the amounts of bowel medication given to their continuing care patients. Emly et al. (1998) directly compared abdominal massage with laxative therapy in a profoundly disabled institutionalised population, and found that the effects of both treatments were not demonstrably different. Emly (1993) has had considerable success with the massage programmes that have been initiated.

Abdominal massage may be performed using just a carrier oil or with the addition of appropriate essential oils. Abdominal massage is best performed using firm effleurage, using the heel of the hand, and should begin in the right iliac fossa and follow the normal route of the gut. The massage may take up to 15 minutes. Suitable essential oils include *Piper ingram*, *Origanum marjorana*, *Rosa damascena*, *Foeniculum vulgare* and *Citrus vulgaris* (orange). A warm compress, using some of these oils applied to the abdomen, may soothe any abdominal pain or colic. Oils such as *Cymbopogum citrates* (lemongrass) and *Salvia officinalis* (sage) could be used to deodorise the environment. Bach flower remedies may be used if an emotional cause is suspected and any reflexology treatment will focus on the intestinal, circulatory and lymphatic points to aid elimination.

A case study of a constipated patient

Trudy, aged 59, still works as a traffic warden. She leads a very busy life and, in the course of a day, because of her job, walks approximately 10 miles. She has a BMI of 22 and a good appetite, eats a well-balanced diet, but tends to eat a lot of cheese. She drinks only socially and smokes 20 cigarettes a day. She has had non-allergic asthma since babyhood and is on Ventolin and Becotide (steroid based) inhalers 4- to 6-hourly and as required.

She presented for treatment because of chronic constipation, which she has suffered for many years. She takes over-the-counter laxatives every night because she feels that her colon is very sluggish. She appears anxious and extremely nervous and is very wheezy. She is post-menopausal, but says that she suffers from mood swings although she did not seek help for this. She has no problems with micturition, but her right shoulder is stiff. She has a ruddy complexion with a fine spotty rash under its surface.

Initial visit

When she walked in I observed some wheeziness in her chest and could smell cigarette smoke on her breath. I chose to use *Origanum marjorana* (marjoram) and *Foeniculum vulgare* for her constipation and possible toxic-ity, and added *Styrax benzoin* for her chestiness plus the uplifting *Pelargonium odorantissimum* (geranium) for her mood swings and skin (I drop of each per 10 ml of base oil). I massaged the backs of her legs and upper chest to aid lymphatic drainage, her abdomen for the constipation, and her face to help her skin and sinuses. I contacted her respiratory and digestive reflex zones on both feet and stimulated her adrenals and solar plexus to alleviate her anxiety. After treatment her nose ran and she felt abdomi-nally bloated. We discussed her diet and I advised that she reduce her cheese intake because of its propensity for mucus formation. She was unsure as to whether she would return but would ring.

Second visit

Trudy did make another appointment because she had felt more relaxed and less sluggish since her therapy. She had reduced her cheese intake and was considering giving up smoking but would need some help with this. As I would be away for a few days I suggested she bought the Bach flower remedy walnut and take as directed to help her 'move herself on'.

She did not return.

Haemorrhoids

Haemorrhoids or piles are varicose veins in the rectum and they normally occur as a result of straining at stool. They may be temporary or permanent and tend to be very painful. As it hurts to defaecate, patients may also become constipated as a result of having haemorrhoids. The two conditions therefore often aggravate each other. They may be soothed by applying essential oils such as *Pogostemon patchouli* (patchouli), *Commiphora myrrha*, *Juniperus communis*, *Cupressus sempervirens* (cypress) and *Boswellia thurifera* locally. They may be added to a sitz bath or applied directly in a cream base or with a wash cloth.

Irritable bowel syndrome

Irritable bowel syndrome (IBS) is a collection of irritating symptoms that make up this syndrome. They include abdominal pain and cramps, diarrhoea, constipation and often flatulence. The sufferer may experience these symptoms separately, but at times may have them all at the same time. There is some evidence that complementary therapies can help this difficult condition. The aim of treatment is to reduce the pain and associated stress and encourage a more conducive way of life (Parker 1999).

Although Mantle (1996) notes that acupuncture and hypnosis have proved helpful, the study of Leahy et al. (1998) suggests that relaxation may also prove beneficial. Out of the 46 patients with untreatable IBS symptoms who were taught progressive relaxation, more than 50% found it to be helpful in relieving these symptoms. Even those whose symptoms were not relieved said that they felt less pain and also that they were more in control. The researchers thought it unlikely that this was the result of a placebo effect because the participants had failed to respond to antispasmodic medication and dietary measures before the study.

Parker (1999) is convinced that regular aromatherapy massage of the abdomen can help such sufferers, especially if it is combined with dietary and lifestyle advice. When treating patients she uses a combination of oils such as *Jasminum officinale* and *Origanum marjorana* for stress and anxiety, *Mentha piperita* and *Zingiber officinale* as a carminative or antispasmodic, and *Pelargonium graveolens* or *Rosa damascena* (rose) for their antidepressant properties. After treatment she advises that they drink warm chamomile tea and apply a warm compress of the same essential oils to help alleviate pain and abdominal spasm. She has found that, once the patients feel in control of their symptoms, they are then ready to embrace changes within their diet and lifestyle, which may then bring further relief.

Complementary therapies have a part to play in the minor problems and symptoms associated with the alimentary tract. As many digestive disorders are emotionally influenced they may also have a role to play in the creation of more harmonious environments, which support such patients.

Learning activity

1. Look at your traditional management of digestive disorders and consider ways in which any of the above strategies may enhance the care that your clients/patients receive.
2. Devise an assessment and evaluation instrument that you could use to inform and appraise the use of complementary approaches in the management of constipation in your client/patient group.

References

Ballard A (1996) Traditional and complementary therapies used together in the treatment, relief and control of Crohn's disease and polyarthritis. Complementary Therapies in Nursing and Midwifery 2: 52–54.

Booth B (1993) Nutritional therapies. Nursing Standard 89(37): 44–46.

Bush S (2000) Fluids, fibre and constipation. NT Plus 96(31): 11–12.

Davis P (1999) Aromatherapy an A–Z, revised edn. Saffron Walden: CW Daniel Co. Ltd.

Emly M (1993) Abdominal massage. Nursing Times 89(3): 34–36.

Emly M, Cooper S, Vail A (1998) Colonic motility in profoundly disabled people: a comparison of massage and laxative therapy in the management of constipation. Physiotherapy 84: 178–183.

Leahy A, Clayman C, Mason I, Lloyd G, Epstein O (1998) Computerised biofeedback games: a new method for teaching stress management and its use in irritable bowel syndrome. Journal of the Royal College of Physicians of London 32: 552–556.

Liu S, Manson J, Stampfer M (2000) Whole grain consumption and risk of ischaemic stroke in women. Journal of the American Medical Association 284: 1534–1540.

Mantle F (1996) Eliminate the problem. Nursing Times 92(32): 50–51.

Madden V (2000) Nutritional benefit of drinks. Nursing Standard 15(13–15): 47–54.

Nazarko L (2000) How age affects fluid intake. NT Plus 96(31): 8.

Parker L (1999) A guide to the use of aromatherapy in irritable bowel syndrome. Aromatherapy World: Nurturing Summer: 18–19.

Reid D (1994) The Tao of Health, Sex and Longevity. London: Simon & Schuster.

Resende T, Brocklehurst J, O'Neill P (1993) A pilot study on the effect of exercise and abdominal massage in continuing care patients. Clinical Rehabilitation 7: 204–209.

Smith-Warner S (2001) Intake of fruits and vegetables and risk of breast cancer. Journal of the American Medical Association 285: 769–776.

Tanner R (1990) Step by Step Reflexology. Surrey: Douglas Barry Pubs.

Thomas S (1992) Eating and drinking. In: Redfern S, ed., Nursing Elderly People. Edinburgh: Churchill Livingstone.

Wasling C (1999) Role of the cardioprotective diet in preventing coronary heart disease. British Journal of Nursing 8: 1239–1248.

Werbach M (1997) A diet for multiple sclerosis. International Journal of Alternative and Complementary Medicine 15(5): 8.

Worwood V (1994) The Fragrant Pharmacy. London: Bantam Books.

Further reading

Brown D (1993) Headway Guides: Aromatherapy. London: Hodder & Stoughton.

Brown D (1993) Headway Guides: Massage. London: Hodder & Stoughton.

Howard J (1990) The Bach Flower Remedies Step by Step. Saffron Walden: CW Daniel Co. Ltd.

Mantle F (1996b) A taste of health. Nursing Times 92(27): 50–51.

Rankin-Box D (2000) An alternative approach to bowel disorders. NT Plus 96(19): 24–26.

Rector-Page L (1996) Controlling Allergies and Overcoming Asthma with Herbs. New York: Healthy Healing Publications.

Richards A (1998) Hands on help. Nursing Times 94(32): 69–75.

Stormer C (1995) Reflexology. The definitive guide. Reading: Hodder & Stoughton.

CHAPTER 10

Genitourinary system

Ageing has a profound effect on the genitourinary system and creates bothersome symptoms and conditions that are often amenable to complementary therapy intervention. Although with advancing age genitourinary problems become quite common, because they involve such personal bodily functions, older people, who have not been brought up to discuss such things openly, find them very difficult to confront. Although many of the problems encountered within these systems are considered quite minor ones, to the individuals themselves they are often catastrophic, especially because patients find them so embarrassing and tedious to live with.

Often patients kep their problems a secret for many years because either they are very ashamed of them or they do not know how to seek help. Therefore when patients do admit that they have a problem and come for treatment, they need to be handled with the utmost respect and, needless to say, should not be offered false hope. This is never truer than when considering sexual problems. The taboo subject of sexuality in the older person will therefore encompass the debate surrounding the problems that arise in sexual expression within elderly people in institutionalised settings.

Consequently this chapter does not involve itself with the treatments of major diseases but instead explores ways in which complementary therapies may either remedy or help patients cope with these symptoms. I have found that it is useful to adopt a combined approach when treating these patients, especially as many of the problems experienced are emotionally influenced.

Frequency and incontinence

Two of the most common problems that older people experience are frequency and incontinence. They may appear as a transient symptom of many illnesses or more probably as a result of a urinary tract infection (UTI). As patients are fearful that they will 'have an accident' because they are unable to control their bladders, they are often reluctant to go out. Without help such sufferers can soon become socially withdrawn and at risk of developing other problems. Although it is sensible for them to increase their fluid intake up to 3000 ml/day, they are often reluctant to do so, because they think it will exacerbate their frequency and incontinence.

Incontinence is a particularly insidious condition because it is socially unacceptable within society to void inappropriately and from an early age we are all taught this. As well as this, if the problem continues patients may experience additional discomforts such as soreness and the embarrassing smell of stale urine. It is essential that all patients with such problems are thoroughly investigated and offered some bladder re-training before adopting other therapies. Complementary therapies may be used as an adjunct to this or as a means of helping them cope longer term. Therapists must be very patient and adopt a non-judgemental approach when dealing with patients who suffer from frequency or incontinence, because any impatience or displeasure will only generate more anxiety within the patient, which will, in turn, further exacerbate the problem.

Essential oils

These are very useful in helping patients cope with continence problems in several ways. They could relieve the following:

- Soreness: a sitz bath containing *Citrus bergamia* (bergamot) and *Santalum album* (sandalwood) for men or *Citrus bergamia* and *Lavandula angustifolia* (lavender) for women.
- Associated negative feelings: *Jasminum officinale* (jasmine) and *Juniperus communis* (juniper).
- Embarrassing odours: deodorising oils include: *Mentha piperita* (peppermint), *Thymus vulgaris* (thyme) and *Salvia officinalis* (sage). For other sweet smelling oils, see Chapter 4.

Flower remedies

These are particularly useful because they help combat the inevitable negative emotions that surface when facing such problems. Many of them would be infinitely suitable. But the ones I have especially chosen are those that will not only help patients deal with their condition but also help them 'move on' and embrace treatment positively. I therefore recommend the following: rock rose, water violet, white chestnut, agrimony, crab apple, gentian and gorse. Patients may also benefit from the composite Rescue Remedy, especially when they are attempting to emerge from the confines of their own home and engage in society once more.

Cystitis

Although cystitis is more often caused by a bacterial infection, irritants within the bladder can also cause this inflammatory condition. Although it is more common in women it can affect men. As you get older the ability to empty the bladder diminishes, because some bladder tone is lost. As a result of this the residual urine, left within the bladder, creates the ideal environment for bacteria to multiply and therefore puts older people more at risk of developing other bladder problems.

Cystitis can be helped by massage and the judicious use of essential oils. The lower abdomen can be massaged very gently with a carrier oil containing a mixture of one or two essential oils. If the abdomen is too tender a hot compress of the same diluted oils could be placed over the symphisis pubis or lower back to bring some relief. These could also be added to a bath. Tisserand (1990) recommends that patients should have a sitz bath every time they void urine wherever possible, especially where dysuria is present. Suitable essential oils include *Citrus bergamia, Lavandula angustifolia, Melaleuca alternifolia* (tea-tree), *Anthemis nobilis* (Roman chamomile), *Juniperus communis* and *Melaleuca leucadendron* (cajuput). I would, wherever possible, include in this blend *Citrus bergamia*, because of its affinity with the urinary tract. Patients should also be advised to drink plenty of water and to consult their doctor if the symptoms persist.

Case study of a patient with cystitis and other symptoms

Roberta was an extremely anxious yet superficially calm, young looking 70-year-old retired headmistress. She was a very private, single woman who was very reticent to speak of the new man in her life, albeit she was obviously sensitive about him, especially as she presented with cystitis. She had suffered from recurrent headaches for several years and often woke, because of this, during the night and then experienced difficulty in getting back to sleep. Her skin was extremely dry. She stated that she was very concerned about her forthcoming driving theory test.

She was reluctant to undress so I just asked her to remove her top, leaving her bra on and propped her up, on her back, on the couch. I spent some time just talking to her. As she disliked the smell of lavender we decided against using it. Into 10 ml of composite carrier oil I added 1 drop of *Salvia sclarea* (clary sage) because it is useful for anxiety and stress but also has a great affinity for the urinary tract. As this also blends well with *Citrus bergamia*, I added 1 drop of this to help both her cystitis and her skin. Finally 1 drop of *Boswellia thurifera* (frankincense) and the Bach flower remedy mimulus was added to reduce her anxiety. I felt that, if I could remedy this overriding problem, then perhaps her insomnia and headaches would resolve. I gently massaged her upper chest to drain her upper lymphatics into her axillae. Then I continued to treat her face and finally massaged the back of her shoulders and scalp. She appeared to relax, somewhat overcoming her fidgety, embarrassed behaviour. I gave her the remaining mixture to bathe in that night and I advised her to drink copious amounts of water. She agreed to return the next day.

Second visit

She said she had not slept very well but felt that her cystitis was a little easier. I did not feel able to discuss her new relationship with her, so I continued as before and gave her the same post-treatment advice. She again agreed to return the next day.

Third visit

She was extremely anxious so I continued as before. I gave her the composite Bach flower Rescue Remedy to take before her test and also enough *Citrus bergamia*, *Salvia sclarea* and *Juniperus communis* (in a solution of 1 drop of each in 10 ml of carrier oil) to bathe in nightly until she returned for treatment.

Fourth visit

Her cystitis had resolved but she was now anxious about the practical driving test. As she had had a very cleansing mixture over the last 2 weeks, I asked her if she would let me also massage her legs, to drain her lower lymphatics. She agreed. As she no longer needed to be so stimulated, I used *Rosa damascena* (rose) and *Anthemis nobilis* to calm her. I continued with the *Citrus bergamia* (1 drop per 10 ml), for her skin and in case there was any residual urinary tract infection. After treatment she was quite relaxed and even chatty. I just asked her to continue to drink and bathe in the remaining oil at night. She agreed to return in 5 days.

Fifth visit

She said her head was not so painful but that she still felt anxious. In addition to the regimen of the fourth visit, I stimulated the adrenal and pituitary reflexes zones of her feet to try to induce some natural stress relief. She was fascinated by this and would return in 1 week.

Sixth visit

As she had found this beneficial I continued as for the fifth visit.

She attended twice more, passed her driving test and is continuing with her new relationship.

> Look again at Chapter 4 and Appendix I and see if you can identify other suitable oils with which to treat the above patient.

Interstitial cystitis: an example of integrated practice

The work that follows started from a chance remark from a post-registration student in the conclusion of her assignment, written for a diploma level complementary health care module. This student, a continence service team leader, noted that her chosen topic was worthy of further development and I agreed with her. She sought my help to do this and the rest is history!

Although interstitial cystitis (not to be confused with cystitis), commonly referred to as IC, has been described as:

> . . . a syndrome characterised by the symptoms of urinary urgency, frequency, nocturia, lower abdominal and perineal pain, in the absence of infection or other known pathology . . .
>
> Mullholland et al. (1990)

it does not really sum up the full extent of the problem that patients may be experiencing, I feel that the following does:

> Imagine that you need to pass urine every 10–20 minutes, day and night, have dysuria, urgency and vulval pain. You are unable to travel, even short distances, sit through a concert and are frightened and embarrassed to visit friends. Your ability to work is hindered by this constant need to be near a toilet and indeed your ability to enjoy family life in all its forms is devastated.
>
> Brett and Barker (1998)

It is not only these distressing symptoms that affect sufferers but also the frustration that comes from the difficulty in establishing a diagnosis. This is compounded by the devastating awareness that to date there is no one known cure that will relieve their distress and that many of the treatments still leave them with disabling symptoms afterwards (Thompson and Christmas 1996)!

It is estimated that 1000 new cases of IC are diagnosed each year in this country alone; however, some experts claim that up to 30% of all women who have recurrent urinary tract infections could indeed be suffering from IC (Lewi 1996). The prevalence of IC within the general population is therefore difficult to estimate. It was claimed by Oravisto, in 1975, that the incidence of IC was 10 cases per 100 000; however, criteria for diagnosis are so variable that it makes statistics difficult to interpret accurately. IC attacks all ages and is not sex specific, although only 10% of all sufferers are men (Miller et al. 1997). Interestingly, IC is found more commonly in Jewish women than in the general female population and is rare in Black populations (Thompson and Christmas 1996).

Although the aetiology and underlying pathology of IC are still unknown and opinions remain varied, it does not have an underlying bacterial cause; diagnosis is normally made by excluding other diseases (Pontari et al. 1997) and is confirmed by cystoscopy and hydrodistension (Brett and Barker 1998). Current conventional management, depending on where the patient is treated, includes: hydrodistension; tricyclic antidepressants; the use of drugs such as dimethyl sulfoxide (DMSO) and heparin which are both instilled into the bladder, or Elmiron (pentosan polysulphate sodium) and sometimes cimetidine, given orally. Other treatments include: surgical initiatives such as augmentation cystoplasty, which involves removing part of the affected bladder and replacing with bowel; urinary diversion; and cystectomy. Patients sometimes become disenchanted with this confusing and unattractive array of treatments, which they may have to endure.

The local support group

This local support group, set up to help these vulnerable patients, has been running for quite some time, meets quarterly and comprises both male and female participants. It was within this group that we sought ways to help them cope better with this illness, by adopting self-management strategies. The focus became one of introducing the clients to both orthodox and complementary treatments. Although several authors, including the national Interstitial Cystitis Support Group (ICSG), encourage the use of alternative or complementary therapies, we found very little specific information to guide us. It appears therefore that complementary medicine is still:

... a marginal activity in the NHS ...

Trevelyan (1998)

and that the introduction of new approaches has largely been left to enthusiastic individuals, who, it seems, are still hampered in their endeavours by both reluctant managers and medical objectors (Trevelyan 1998). Many of these clients were already disenchanted with and had developed negative attitudes towards their consultants, and we were conscious not to inflame this already tense situation. We were also very careful not to diminish the credibility of other professionals, including other continence advisers who may have different remits for service (Brett and Barker 1998). As it is, this role is widely misunderstood, e.g. the continence adviser is often addressed as:

... the 'incontinent nurse' or 'the pad lady'.

We were keen not to introduce these group participants to poorly researched initiatives or offer false hope because to do so would be unethical. Rankin-Box (1991) suspects that nurses may be using therapies in the belief that they help their clients, even though there is little or no empirical evidence to support this belief. And although Freshwater (1996) feels that it is very sensible for nurses to be cautious when embarking on different care approaches, she feels that there is also a danger of discounting anecdotal information, which may help patients just because it has never been researched quantifiably.

As we were unsure about how to progress, we consulted the literature and found two useful and informative studies (Webster and Brennan 1995, Mendelowitz and Moldwin 1997). Webster and Brennan (1995) found that these sufferers (women only in this study) had:

... used a wide variety of psychological and physical self care strategies, and the most effective of these appeared to be: wearing loose clothing; localised heat applications; some dietary restrictions and to a lesser extent massage, imagery and relaxation tapes. They also noted that because there was so little agreement about the cause and treatment of IC it was extremely hard to decide which of these alternative strategies could be usefully employed.

Brett and Barker (1998)

Mendelowitz and Moldwin's (1997) study found that relaxation and behaviour modification was useful with IC patients. After experiencing face-to-face instruction on the use of their individually designed audiotapes, 76% of the participants reported that it had helped their urological condition, another 43% felt that it helped their other medical conditions and 93% would recommend their use to other sufferers.

As others (Reid Czarapata 1994) and our group members themselves had discussed the potential of relaxation with us, we investigated how we could realistically introduce such tapes. Although massage had been identified as a complementary treatment option, the extra time and resources involved currently preclude this. We felt that relaxation tapes were especially pertinent for this group because, carefully designed, they could go some way to replacing the therapist and could be used wherever they were.

Before embarking on this, you need, however, to consider the initial outlay involved, although often you find that many patients/clients already have access to portable stereo-recorders. Although these are ideal because they are so light, some of the dials may be difficult for older patients to manage, because either they have lost some of the fine pincer movements in their hands or their sight is too poor for them to see them clearly. If patients do not possess their own stereos and are thinking of purchasing one, it is useful to warn them about this.

Careful consideration must also be given to the actual design of the audiotapes that are used, so that patients can benefit from them. When doing this it may be useful to consider Table 10.1.

To recap, audio relaxation tapes and music are a means of providing the patient with some distraction from their treatment (O'Sullivan 1991), and they are extremely useful because their use can be continued by the patient at home (McGourty and Hotchkiss 1993). This, in turn, may give the patients greater control over their condition and also has the potential to aid their own recovery.

The group is still meeting regularly and we have found, like Feinmann (1997), that it is helping them to cope with their disease and also manage some of their symptoms because it allows them access to 'expert' advice and discussion of their problems in a friendly and equal relationship. It also allows them to 'sound off', about past interventions, in a safe and secure haven. The ICSG appear to have used this approach for several years and we acknowledge their work. Amazingly Skene, at the Royal London Hospital, first described IC over 125 years ago but it appears that we are only now beginning to make significant progress in the understanding of its cause and treatments (Christmas 1997).

Can you differentiate between cystitis and interstitial cystitis?
As IC is currently not curable what are the potential dangers of introducing patients to the notion of using alternative approaches?

Table 10.1 Choosing a tape

1. Choose a relaxation tape that includes both visualisation advice and music. Research shows that there is an increased efficiency in the level of relaxation when it is combined with visualisation and during trials a significant number of people expressed a preference to listening to a sound while experiencing a therapy, rather than just silence (Kneafsey 1997). The most popular sounds reported were music of their own choice, the sea and a waterfall (Garnett 1994). Therefore it would be beneficial to choose relaxation tapes for the patients that included both visualisation and music. Ryman (1994) warns that the tapes should not trigger any adverse emotions in the client, e.g. it may be inappropriate to ask a patient with hay fever to visualise a cornfield. Good (1995) suggests that patients should be encouraged to use techniques that they have found beneficial in the past, especially if they are reluctant to engage in this activity. Patients must be warned that any new pain or discomfort should be reported while using these techniques.

2. Use music with the correct pitch, tempo and volume. Listening to soothing music appears to induce a hypometabolic response which, in turn, helps reduce heart rate and may afford greater pain relief because it is thought to increase an individual's pain threshold (Guzetta 1989) The tempo of 70–80 beats/min appears to be the most calming, because it seems to reduce tension. Loud and high-pitched music should be avoided, because it tends to increase tension and may even cause pain (O'Sullivan 1991). The music needs to be tailored to each patient's needs and it would seem that the music of choice should be slow with a steady rhythm of low frequency, melodious and familiar (Cook 1986).

3. The tapes should be designed so that the music is not continuous and become a nuisance, but be interspersed with relaxation and visualisation sessions throughout (O'Sullivan 1991), because there is some evidence that such measures can influence physiological change and psychological well-being (Ryman 1994), albeit some of the findings relating to patients' well-being are deemed to be subjective (Burke and Sikora 1992). If, however, pain is considered to be what the patient says it is, why is it that the same claims cannot be made about general well-being (Tattam 1992)?

4. The tape needs to be personalised and reflect individual symptoms and not just the non-specific symptoms associated generally with all IC sufferers. Its design must also consider when it is appropriate to include muscle relaxation, pain management and stress reduction exercises or only some of them (Mendelowitz and Moldwin 1997). Although there are few reported contraindications with using tapes, there may be potential problems if the patient has considerable abdominal pain. In this instance it would be preferable if the tape focused only on general relaxation because techniques that encourage alternate flexing and relaxing of muscles may exacerbate this. One of the biggest advantages of purposeful relaxation and visualisation is that it helps clients not only to come to terms with their condition but also to rid themselves of the negative connotations associated with their disease (Ryman 1994). One study has also suggested that used together they provide a more effective treatment than just relaxation alone (Garnett 1994).

5. It is imperative to have initial face-to-face contact when instructing the client in how to use these effectively, preferably in a quiet environment, with the appropriate apparatus, such as personal stereos and headphones available.

6. The tapes need to be cost-effective of time and money and be effective.
   We are currently at this stage of development.

Sexuality and older people

Although there may be a decline in sexual energy in both sexes, some interest and activity in sexual relationships persist for many older people through the late decades, albeit any response may be slower and less intense. The need for intimacy and affection should be accepted and never ridiculed, and it is essential that we recognise that being able to express sexuality is still a very important part of an older person's life. It may be easier to accept this if we remember that sexuality does not just relate to intimacy, but encompasses all the:

> ... sociocultural, psychological and ethical components of sexual behaviour.
>
> (Brogan 1996)

Yet, often, any sexual activity is regarded as inappropriate for older people to engage in, especially by carers who are poorly educated and may also have been socially conditioned into denying the needs of such patients (Webb 1987, Rafferty 1995). It seems that, although carers have a more liberal view of their own sexual activity, they often appear to have unrealistic expectations of older people (Jones 1994). Services are therefore not geared to allow sexual expression or even any discussion about anything remotely sexual. This is often compounded by the fact that older people are regarded as asexual beings, especially where they display physical and/or mental infirmities (Smook 1992)

Although practitioners of complementary therapies cannot alter such perceptions, by attempting to treat such patients in a more holistic way, it may alter some of the current negative stereotypical attitudes surrounding this aspect of care. It must be recognised that carers may need to help older people adopt appropriate strategies so that their sexual needs may be met. Although this may be relatively easy, within the patient's own home, it may be very troublesome within institutionalised settings, because historically they have impeded such activities. Often, sexual inactivity is imposed and is commonly caused by bereavement, impaired mobility (Parke 1991) or drug-induced impotence (Wheeler 1990).

When reviewing a new publication by the Relatives' and Residents' Association, which stated that nurses were not sensitive to the needs of institutionalised elderly people, O'Dowd (2001) noted the depth of feeling that the book elicited! It highlighted several inadequacies, including those that related to meeting the sexual needs of these residents. It seems that this was compounded by a lack of privacy and the resentment of some relatives who felt discouraged from participating more fully in their relative's care. The response to this argument was that nurses were trying very hard to fulfil these obligations but, in a stretched service with dwindling resources, it was just another demand that they found hard to satisfy.

Although there is little research into this subject, it does seem that many of the problems may arise because patient assessments and much of the very intimate care given to older adults are still being carried out by very young women who are often somewhat embarrassed by this (Platzer 1990, Smook 1992).

Although there is a considerable amount of literature, both anecdotal and otherwise, written on the complementary treatments for sexual problems experienced by women, there is very little available to guide the treatment of men.

The ageing woman

Most female sexual changes occur as a result of a reduction in their sex hormones. Ovulation and menstruation cease and the uterus, vagina, genitals and breasts atrophy. The vaginal secretions become less acid and as a consequence of this the mucosa becomes thinner and drier and more easily irritated. This increases the risk of vaginal inflammation and infection.

The menopause and postmenopausal problems

Although every woman's experience of the menopause is likely to be different, there are some essential oils that are particularly useful at this time and a selection are presented below:

- *Rosa damascena* because it acts as a uterine tonic (Mantle 1996) and cleanser and also makes a woman feel more desirable (Hopkins 1995). It is also excellent for older skin (Davis 1999).
- *Foeniculum vulgare* (fennel) for its oestrogenic properties.
- *Salvia sclarea* for its oestrogenic properties and ability to balance extreme emotions, reduce stress and restore inner tranquillity. It is therefore eminently suitable for the alleviation of menopausal difficulties. It is also widely believed to be able to induce a state of euphoria and act as an aphrodisiac, and it blends well with *Santalum album*, *Rosa damascena* and *Anthemis nobilis*, although it is especially useful in combination with *Pelargonium graveolens* because of its ability to balance hormones effectively, especially at the time of the menopause. It also acts as a diuretic so is helpful where fluid retention is a problem.

- *Commiphora myrrha* (myrrh) where fungal infections are troublesome.
- *Citrus aurantium* for its ability to calm, reduce anxiety and depression, and therefore lift emotions.
- *Cananga odorata* (ylang ylang) because it is said to calm anger, release tension, lift depression and generally stabilise mood swings. It is known in Asia as an aphrodisiac (Hopkins 1995).

Hormone replacement therapy

Where women are unable or reluctant to be treated with hormone replacement therapy (HRT), they may be helped by *Foeniculum vulgare* to boost the lowered oestrogen levels after the menopause. As it is a member of the Umbelliferae family, it contains anethol, which has oestrogen-like properties. Sclareol present in *Salvia sclarea* also has this property. Davis (1999) recommends that these oils are not used long term, but just to give a 'kick start' to treatment. She also notes that oestrogen should be balanced with progesterone at this time, but, as no essential oils contain progesterone, patients should be advised to take herbs such as *Vitus agnus-castus* or lady's mantle to supplement this. Fennel is also available as a herbal tea to drink.

Bach flower remedies and reflexology

There are two Bach flower remedies that are particularly indicated for the menopause. Walnut is very useful because it enables women not only to embrace the various changes that are happening but also to move forward positively. Olive, on the other hand, is very effective because of its restorative properties so often needed to combat the physical and emotional fatigue sometimes experienced (Brown 1993b). A generalised reflexology treatment can also help to re-establish the physical, hormonal and emotional balance at this time

Frigidity

See below under Impotence.

Thrush and pruritis

These are both amenable to treatment by bathing with essential oils. Some recommend the use of douches (Tisserand 1990, Worwood 1994) but I would be reluctant to advise this. Davis (1999) also urges caution in this because of the potential dangers of using concentrated essential oils on delicate mucous membranes.

The fungal infection thrush affects all mucous membranes in both men and women. The most appropriate aromatherapy treatment for vaginal thrush is a bath, into which has been added antifungal essential oils such as *Commiphora myrrha*, *Lavandula angustifolia* and *Melaleuca alternifolia*, either singly or as a blend of all three. The same treatment could be used on men whose genitalia are affected by thrush. Pruritis or itching of the mucous membranes responds well to the soothing and anti-inflammatory *Anthemis nobilis* and *Lavandula angustifolia*. They may be added to a bath. If pruritis is caused by a fungal infection, antifungal oils will obviously also be required. If patients are unable to get into a bath, the same solution could be used for washing the area. Other investigations may need to be made and extra advice given about diet and hygiene if these problems keep occurring.

Often people seek treatment for the above minor irritations but also for symptoms that are personally displeasing to them. In my experience swollen ankles are an example of this.

Fluid retention

Fluid retention and oedema may occur for a variety of reasons and should always be properly investigated in case it masks serious illness. It does, however, seem to be a problem that many experience. It responds well to localised massage, especially when essential oils with diuretic properties are used. The massage needs to be firm and should aim to drain the fluid into the nearest lymph nodes. I have found *Cupressus sempervirens* (cypress) to be particularly effective but would also recommend *Citrus limonum* (lemon), *Pelargonium graveolens*, *Rosemarinus officinalis* (rosemary), *Eucalyptus globulus* (eucalyptus) and *Santalum album*. Patients could also use a combination of these added to a bath or as a body rub.

Reflexology

Reflexology is also very effective in reducing swelling and I often combine it with the above aromatherapy massage. After a cursory exploration of the reflex zones, I would then concentrate on the reflexes of the affected areas and the circulatory, lymphatic and urinary reflexes to help eliminate the excess fluid.

An example of treatment given to one of my patient's with swollen ankles

Fiftynine-year-old Marlene had quite a few medical problems. She was on medication for arthritis and asthma and was also on HRT for her postmenopausal problems. But the problem she was most troubled about was her hugely swollen ankles. As a result of all her medication, I was cautious in the oils I chose. To 15 ml of carrier oil I added 1 drop each of *Anthemis nobilis, Citrus limonum, Foeniculum vulgare* and *Lavandula angustifolia*. I gave her a complete aromatherapy massage and drained her legs and ankles using lymphatic drainage, similar to very firm effleurage. At the end of the first session her ankles were much less swollen and her shoes were loose.

She attends regularly each week for the same maintenance treatment because both she and her husband find it cosmetically pleasing that her ankles are less stout.

A favourite blend

A favourite combination of essential oils of mine is *Anthemis nobilis, Pelargonium graveolens, Rosa damascena, Foeniculum vulgare,* and *Cupressus sempervirens* because I have found it very useful as a standby for most 'female problems'. It can be added to a bath, used as a body rub and vaporised or spritzed into the atmosphere to create a calming and uplifting environment.

The ageing male

Reproductive ability persists to a much later age in the male because atrophy of the testicles occurs at a later age than atrophy of the ovaries. The older male may, however, experience hypertrophy of the prostate gland, which can lead to difficulty in voiding and incomplete emptying of the bladder.

Prostatitis

The ageing prostate is also susceptible to inflammation and prostatitis may be acute or chronic and caused by many different reasons, which should be investigated. Massage of the lower abdomen and back may reduce the pain and associated heaviness and bathing in comforting diluted essential oils can alleviate the burning sensation when voiding. Worwood (1994) suggests a combination of lavender, cypress, *Eucalyptus radiata* and thyme linalool to be used three times a day.

Impotence

As there is often no physical cause for impotence, the underlying anxiety, which often accompanies this diagnosis, may respond very well to complementary approaches. Tanner (1990) advocated that, within the complete reflexology treatment regimen, for clients with impotence the following reflex points should be stimulated: solar plexus, pituitary, brain, thyroid and parathyroid glands, testicles, prostate, spleen and the lymphatics. You will note that her emphasis is not only on the physical zones concerned but also very much on those associated with stress and anxiety.

Aromatherapy is also useful because the oils have the potential to act as an aphrodisiac. Oils that are eminently suitable include *Santalum album*, *Zingiber officinale* (ginger) and *Jasminum officinale*. Where there is deep-rooted anxiety *Citrus aurantium* and *Salvia sclarea* are very useful. Oils may be added to a bath before retiring for the night to aid relaxation, or they may be diluted in a carrier oil and massaged into the skin. Initially the judicious use of asexual touch may encourage the client to relax. After a while, it may be appropriate to teach the patient's partner some relaxing massage techniques, stressing all the time that they are not purely intended to act as a precursor for sex.

Reflexology

Stormer (1995) advocates that both partners should be treated. His reflexology regimen includes a generalised treatment of the digestive system reflexes and the liver. Extra attention is given to the following: the central nervous system and solar plexus reflexes to boost confidence and reduce frustration; the endocrines to re-establish emotional control; the reproductive organs to release tension; and the circulatory, lymphatic and urinary systems to re-energise.

Frigidity

For women who are frigid, Stormer (1995) recommends much the same treatment, because the prime aim is to help them to become more open to self-love and responsive within a caring relationship. Women may also be helped in this by the other advice given under impotence, although the more female-type essential oils such as *Rosa damascena*, *Pelargonium grave-olens* and *Cananga odorata* may be preferred.

It is quite clear that many of the above symptoms are both very embarrassing and difficult for patients to live with and, although complementary therapies are not able to cure most of them, they are able to provide considerable relief. They are helpful in alleviating not only some of the physical symptoms but also the associated anxieties. Used wisely they may encourage a more open and courageous approach for sufferers when embracing treatment.

References

Brett H, Barker S (1998) Beating the burn. Nursing Times **94**(32): 75–79.

Brogan M (1996) The sexual needs of elderly people: addressing the issue. Nursing Standard **10**(24): 42–45.

Brown D (1993b) Headway Guides: Massage. London: Hodder & Stoughton .

Bush S (2000) Fluids, fibre and constipation. NT Plus **96**(31): 11–12.

Burke D, Sikora K (1992) Cancer: the dual approach. Nursing Times **88**(38): 63–66.

Christmas T (1997) Historical Aspects of Interstitial Cystitis. Interstitial Cystitis. Philadelphia, PA: Lippincott-Raven.

Cook J (1986) Music as an intervention in the oncology setting. Cancer Nursing **9**(1): 23–28.

Davis P (1999) Aromatherapy an A–Z, revised edn. Saffron Walden: CW Daniel Co. Ltd.

Feinmann J (1997) Fellow travellers. Nursing Times **93**(42): 44–45.

Freshwater D (1996) Complementary therapies and research in nursing practice. Nursing Standard **10**(38): 43–45.

Garnett M (1994) Sounding it out. Nursing Times **90**(34): 64–68.

Good M (1995) Relaxation techniques for surgical patients. American Journal of Nursing **5**: 39–43.

Guzetta C (1989) Effects of relaxation therapy on patients in a CCU with presumptive MI. Heart and Lung **18**: 609–616.

Hopkins C (1995) Aromatherapy: Remedies for Everyday Ailments. Bristol: Parallel Books.

Jones H (1994) Mores and morals. Nursing Times **90**(47): 55–59.

Kneafsey R (1997) The therapeutic use of music in a care of the elderly setting: a literature review. Journal of Clinical Nursing **6**: 341–346.

Lewi H (1996) Family Circle Magazine. April.

McGourty H, Hotchkiss J (1993) Study Rules. Nursing Times **89**(36): 425.

Mantle F (1996) Altered states. Nursing Times **92**(40): 48–49.

Mendelowitz F, Moldwin R (1997) complementary approaches in the management of interstitial cystitis. In: Interstitial Cystitis. Philadelphia, PA: Lippincott-Raven.

Miller J, Bavendam T, Berger T (1997) Interstitial cystitis in men. Interstitial Cystitis. Philadelphia, PA: Lippincott-Raven.

Mullholland SG, Hanno P, Parsons CL, Sant GR, Staskin DR (1990) Pentosan polysulfate sodium for therapy of interstitial cystitis. Urology **35**: 552–558.

O'Dowd A (2001) It's that old devil called love. Nursing Times **97**(17): 13.

Oravisto K (1975) Epidemiology of interstitial cystitis. Annales Chirurgiae et Gynaecologiae (Helsinki) **64**: 75–77.

O'Sullivan R (1991) A musical road to recovery: music in intensive care. Intensive Care Nursing **7**: 160–163.

Parke F (1991) Sexuality in later life. Nursing Times **87**(50): 40–42.

Platzer H (1990) Sexual orientation: improving care. Nursing Standard **4**(38): 38–39.

Pontari M et al. (1997) Logical and systematic approach to the evaluation and management of patients suspected of having interstitial cystitis. Urology **49**(suppl 5A): 114–120.

Rafferty D (1995) Putting sexuality on the agenda. Nursing Times **91**(17): 28–31.

Rankin-Box D (1991) Proceed with caution. Nursing Times **87**(45): 34–36.

Reid Czarapata B (1994) Clinical highlights: management of interstitial cystitis. Urological Nursing **14**: 145–148.

Ryman L (1994) Relaxation and visualisation. In: Wells R, Tschudin V, eds, Wells' Supportive Therapies in Health Care. London: Baillière Tindall.

Smook K (1992) Nurses' attitudes toward the sexuality of older people: an investigative study. Nursing Practice **6**(1): 15–17.

Stormer C (1995) Reflexology. The definitive guide. Reading: Hodder & Stoughton.

Tanner R (1990) Step by Step Reflexology. Surrey: Douglas Barry.

Tattam A (1992) The gentle touch. Nursing Times **88**(32): 16–17.

Thompson A, Christmas T (1996) Interstitial cystitis – an update. British Journal of Urology **78**: 813–820.

Tisserand M (1990) Aromatherapy for Women. London: Thorsons.

Trevelyan J (1998) Complementary Options. Nursing Times **94**(13): 28–29.

Webb C (1987) Sexual healing. Nursing Times **83**(32): 29–30.

Webster D, Brennan T (1995) Self-care strategies used for acute attack of Interstitial Cystitis. Urologic Nursing 15(3): 86–93.

Wheeler V (1990) A new kind of loving? Professional Nurse June: 492–496.

Worwood V (1994) The Fragrant Pharmacy. London: Bantam Books.

Further reading

Howard J (1990) The Bach Flower Remedies Step by Step. Saffron Walden: CW Daniel Co. Ltd.

Ingham E (1991) The original works of Eunice D. Ingham. Stories the feet can tell thru reflexology – Stories the feet have told thru reflexology (with revisions by Dwight C Byers). St Petersburg, FL: Ingham Publishing, Inc.

Slade D, Ratner V, Chairir R et al. (1997) A collaborative approach to managing interstitial cystitis. Urology **49**(suppl 5A): 10–13.

CHAPTER 11
Mobility problems

Loss of mobility is common in ageing individuals and there are varying reasons for this. These may include functional and physical losses, disorders of gait and balance, psychosocial factors, hormonal and dietary effects, and also the presence of specific disease. The level and type of immobility also vary and may range from minimal dysfunction to total incapacity. As it is considered normal to experience a general slowing down and some functional change as one ages, even when individuals experience some difficulties they do not consider that they are ill or disabled (Batehup and Squires 1992). I would suspect that a high percentage of patients seek complementary and alternative treatments for relief of pain and stiffness that often accompanies any immobility.

During the ageing process bones become more brittle and there is a reduction in both organic material and osteocytes. In addition to this, there is some demineralisation usually as a result of a reduction of endocrine secretions, such as oestrogen. As a result of these changes in bone structure, there is an increased risk of the incidence of fractures in older people, and joint movement is often restricted and painful because of the degeneration of the cartilage at the ends of weight-bearing bones. Osteoarthritis and rheumatoid arthritis are both common and frequently cause inactivity and immobility in patients. The response rate in the muscles, resulting from atrophy, is normally reduced but less so if the patients remain active. Such disuse of the muscles can lead to fatty infiltration and marked weakness. This may be further aggravated if the patient is obese (see Chapter 9) and takes little or no exercise.

Complementary therapies tend to follow a more holistic approach to care and this approach is very important, because the physical and psychological ramifications of chronic and degenerative diseases are immense. Although the therapies themselves may not cure, they have an important role to play in the daily management of their pain and symptoms. This chapter therefore looks at some of the ways that may help patients regain some control of their own treatments and help them cope with the inevitability of their disease progression.

Massage is extremely useful in chronic conditions because when muscles receive an increased blood supply of nutrients their functioning is improved and waste products that accumulate in muscles, such as uric acid, can also be eliminated. This helps to prevent soreness and aching, and often minimises calf cramps and other muscle spasms. Massage can therefore be used as a form of passive exercise that can partially compensate for lack of exercise and, by improving muscle tone, muscular atrophy, caused by forced inactivity, may be reduced. Massage therapy appears also to relieve pain and many of the other physical and psychological symptoms that patients have to endure.

Essential oils are very useful for such patients because of the various therapeutic properties that they possess and the affinity they have for specific conditions. The ones that are especially efficacious are the analgesic and anti-inflammatory oils (see Appendix I). Reflexology is also extremely helpful because it can aid the elimination of toxins such as uric acid, rebalance and assist pain relief (Tanner 1990, Stormer 1995). Bach flower remedies are also worth considering, because there is often associated negativity with most chronic conditions (Howard 1990).

Rheumatic disease

The social and economic impact of rheumatic diseases, particularly rheumatoid arthritis, is huge because long-term medical care is extremely expensive and often difficult to access. In addition to this, many of the drugs administered to control symptoms and disability have potential side effects, which worry patients. The Arthritis Research Campaign (ARC 2000) felt that, as there was no cure for arthritis, complementary therapies could have a part to play in encouraging patients to adopt positive lifestyle changes that might help to stabilise or improve their individual condition.

Rheumatoid arthritis

As rheumatoid arthritis is a chronic, inflammatory condition that affects all the joints of the body, it responds very well to massage (see Chapter 3 for massage movements) with or without the use of essential oils (see Chapter 4). Patients can experience a good deal of relief from regular massage because it can help 'loosen' and relax individual joints. It is, however, essential to remember that many of these patients will have some permanent joint changes, which restricts their range of movement so that, when trying to release the joints, any movement should not be forced and cause further damage or pain.

Although there has been very little research into the use of massage and/or aromatherapy with rheumatoid patients, and many of the studies are inconclusive (Cawthorne 1991, Brownfield 1998), Vickers (1996) noted that there was some evidence that massage reduced muscle tension and increased blood circulation. He also noted that some of the essential oils did appear to have the potential to alleviate pain and inflammation. Many other authors offer anecdotal advice about such treatment (Say 1991, Brown 1993a, 1993b, *Arthritis News* 1995, Price and Price 1995, Davis 1999). I have found that petrissage around the joints, preceded and followed by effleurage, are two very useful massage strokes not only to aid pain relief but also to mobilise the joints. Patients with osteoarthritis can also benefit from these strokes.

The case study below indicates how essential oils, massage and reflexology were used to help one arthritic sufferer.

Case study

Initial visit

Sally is an obese woman with very limited mobility. As a result of this I had great difficulty getting her on to the couch and was assisted in this by her daughter. She is a 69-year-old housewife who leads a sedentary lifestyle. She smokes but does not drink. She has suffered from rheumatoid arthritis for about 35 years and is on naproxen 250 mg three times a day for her arthritis. She also takes occasional paracetamol for joint pain and swelling, in addition to the naproxen. She is primarily concerned about her arthritis, generalised immobility and restricted walking. She also suffers from severe muscular pain and deformity as a result of her arthritis and possibly her obesity. Her hip, knee and ankle joints are the most troublesome. The arthritic nodules on her fingers cause pain and difficulties with fine movements.

Her diet is very poor because it is high in refined carbohydrate and fat. She drinks several cups of sweet milky tea during the night and during the day snacks on biscuits and tea. She suffers from very occasional indigestion but receives no treatment for this. She takes two Mogadon tablets nightly for insomnia because she sleeps only for short periods and wakes several times during the night. As she is often awake, she gets up to micturate during the night. She has a clear English rose complexion.

A research study by Macdonald (1995) revealed very good results in the relief not only of arthritic pain but also of the associated immobility and insomnia. As Sally fitted all three categories I decided to try the same formula of oils. Unfortunately the study did not specify the genus. I therefore used *Eucalyptus globulus* (eucalyptus), *Juniperus communis* (juniper), *Origanum marjorana* (marjoram) and *Rosemarinus officinalis* (rosemary). Macdonald (1995) advocated that the oils were topically applied twice a day, without massage, in a 1. 5% solution for 10 weeks. We decided that I would apply the treatment each morning for 7 days and that the daughter would apply it in the evening. She was to continue with her medication.

Second visit

At the end of this first week Sally's progress was discussed by all three of us. She felt that the pain and also the immobility were marginally better. She felt that she could continue with this treatment at home because it was hard for her daughter to keep bringing her. I made up the appropriate solution for her. The daughter said she would keep a diary of any changes and that if they needed help she would contact me. We negotiated for Sally to return in 1 month.

Third visit

She reported that her pain was really much easier but her hips felt very stiff. As I was not trying to replicate the study, I decided to apply firm massage to her pelvic girdle and hip joints and also contact the corresponding and cross-reflexes in her feet. After treatment her hips felt less stiff and she was very relaxed. She would continue with the application of oils and return in 1 week.

Fourth visit

She looked very bright and her walking was a little improved She had omitted her night sedation for two nights and slept. Her daughter seemed to think she had lost weight. The scales revealed that she had lost 1 kg. Sally was very pleased and treatment continued as per her last visit. She was advised to continue with her home treatments and return in 2 weeks. She continues to use this blend at home and to reduce the stiffness in her hip joints, and visits every 6 weeks for a back and pelvic massage.

Generalised aches and pains

These are probably the most common conditions that patients present with. Currently I have several patients who, after an initial combined treatment, which may include massage, reflexology and the use of essential oils, feel able to treat themselves at home. Self-treatment may also benefit conditions such as fibrositis, sciatica and fibromyalgia, especially where patients are reluctant to rely on prescription drugs.

Patient examples

Patient 1

A 75-year-old woman with arthritic hands and knees, who also happens to be a colleague's mother, manages to remain pain and stiffness free by the twice-daily application of the following blend. To 25 ml of grapeseed oil are added 3 drops each of *Lavandula angustifolia* (lavender), *Styrax benzoin* (benzoin) and *Piper nigrum* (black pepper), which are all warming and possess analgesic properties, *Anthemis nobilis* (Roman chamomile) for its anti-inflammatory properties and *Rosemarinus officinalis*, which is very useful for arthritic pain. Although she has never been advised to stop taking her prescribed drugs, she has decided that she no longer needs to take any anti-inflammatory or analgesic medication.

Patient 2

A 77-year-old woman, who presented with arthritic hands and shoulders, very painful knees and swollen ankles, has managed not only to relieve her pain but also to reduce the oedema in her ankles. She is very pleased with the results and maintains her treatment by self-massage of the affected parts twice daily. As riding in a car also aggravates her shoulder pain, applying the oils half an hour before travelling gives her tremendous relief. Her blend is made up of 50 ml of grapeseed oil, into which is added 5 drops each of *Piper nigrum* (black pepper), *Anthemis nobilis* (Roman chamomile) and *Rosemarinus officinalis*, *Citrus limonum* (lemon), for the oedema, and *Mentha piperita* (peppermint), for its analgesic properties. As a result of this, the patient no longer has to rely on her codeine-based analgesia and is pleased that her constipation has resolved.

Patient 3

Although she is 62, this woman continues to work in a very demanding job. She presented, approximately 5 years ago, with severe and regular migraines. On examination she was found to be very anxious, have an old neck injury that still troubled her and an allergy to cream. As a result of this I blended 20 ml of grapeseed oil with 2 drops each of *Salvea sclarea* (clary sage) for stress, *Mentha piperita*, to act as an analgesic and also for her digestive problems, and *Lavandula angustifolia*. I also advised her to consider her diet. She applies this mix to her temples and wrists twice daily and, apart from on one occasion, has remained pain and migraine free and no longer has to resort to anti-migrainal medication.

Patient 4

Another woman in her 60s continues to work as a local authority carer on the twilight shift. She presented with neck and lower back pain. She had felt a 'twinge' at work and she sought my help approximately 1 year later! She was advised to seek medical attention for this but has declined to do so. A full body massage immediately eased her neck pain and she continues to use the following essential oils to maintain her lower back pain relief. Into 20 ml of grapeseed oil are added 2 drops each of the following: *Piper nigrum*, *Lavandula angustifolia*, *Anthemis nobilis* and *Zingiber officinalis* (ginger) because it is so warming.

Falls

Our Healthier Nation (Department of Health 1998) states that accidents such as falls are an influential cause of disability and, after experiencing a fall, older people commonly lose their confidence and become less active, socially isolated, lonely and depressed (Castell 1999). In turn, this can lead to a pattern of decreased mobility, flexibility and strength. It is essential therefore that decline in overall function should be delayed as long as possible, thus allowing older adults to live with greater independence and autonomy, and hopefully still be able to experience some quality of life.

Several studies have implicated lower limb muscle weakness as one of the major risk factors in those who fall and Simpson (1993) also suggested that older people who fall may have even weaker muscles than those who do not. It seems that this is especially true of those patients who, because of proximal muscle strength loss, have difficulty in getting up from a chair. Therefore maintaining or improving any muscle strength in an older person may well prolong their independent living (Vitti et al. 1993). Although I could find nothing within the literature that specifically advocated the use of complementary therapies with such patients, as either a preventive or curative measure, because there is evidence to suggest that improved strength, gait and balance lead to improvements in mobility and overall physical activity, it would undoubtedly be useful to investigate whether massage has a role to play in this, passively or otherwise.

Williamson et al. (1987) and Williams and Nolan (1993) have all stressed that patients on prescribed medication, such as diuretics, antidepressants and tranquillisers, are especially at risk of falling, and Marr and Kershaw (1998) have identified that because the common chronic diseases associated with old age, such as arthritis, heart, chest and neurological conditions, often cause physical decline, they can also contribute to falling. As a result of these two reasons, it may be eminently sensible to look at more natural ways of treatment which could reduce the need for medication or other aggressive treatments! (Please see Chapter 12 for an example of using essential oils instead of sedation in a frail, arthritic, nursing home resident.)

Stroke and hemiplegia

Although I recognise that stroke and its associated conditions have a neurological basis, muscle contractures, deformities and restricted joint movement can develop rapidly in such older patients. There is some evidence to suggest that stroke survivors and their relatives seek complementary therapies to meet their longer-term needs, and it seems that dietary measures, acupuncture and massage were the most relevant to them (Johnson et al. 1997). I have found that hand massage, using essential oils such as *Lavandula angustifolia* and *Anthemis nobilis*, are useful in helping to reverse or prevent contractures. Massage to larger muscle groups may also inhibit muscular wasting, although Watson (1997) warns that, if you manipulate joints where there is reduced tone in their stabilising muscles too vigorously, subluxation of the joint could occur. You would also have to exercise caution where there is little or no feeling in a limb, etc.

Back pain

This is also a common complaint and one that needs to be thoroughly investigated before treatment and I have included a case study (below) showing one approach to its treatment.

Case study of a patient with back pain

Initial visit

June is an attractive, confident, 75-year-old obese woman. Her posture is very poor and she walks with a swaying gait and appears to be 'knock-kneed' as she walks on the inner aspects of both feet. Her current problems include chronic back pain, for which she takes DF118 most days. She is also bothered by her excess weight. Her diet is high in protein and carbohydrate and her appetite is good.

Visual examination Both feet were generally pink, with reddened areas along the spinal regions and there were the beginnings of bilateral hallux valgus in both feet. There were operational scars on the outer aspects of both ankles. Her feet were warm to the touch but smelt 'cheesy'. On examination she was tender along the spinal columns, radiating into the hip and lower back areas. Special attention was given to these areas and the cross-reflex to the hip, so the shoulder was also stimulated and the adrenals were contacted to encourage natural pain relief. Generalised massage was given to encourage release of toxins, a 'fishy' smell is indicative of this, and promote increased nerve ending activity.

After treatment June stated she had enjoyed the treatment. I advised her to drink plenty of water to aid toxin release and also to try to adopt a better gait. I explained she needed to walk with even pressure on both of her feet rather than mainly on the medial aspects.

Second visit

Visually her feet looked very similar to the first visit and her posture and gait were still poor. She remained tender along the spinal column, so I continued the treatment as before. After treatment she was relaxed and I again advised her about her walking.

Third visit

June was evidently trying to improve her walking. She had bought new shoes, which seemed to support her feet more, but she still displayed a swaying gait. As the spinal areas of the medial aspects of both feet were red, I concentrated on these. In addition, I stimulated the solar plexus and adrenals to aid natural pain relief, and also massaged the digestive organs because of her obesity and poor diet. I manipulated her feet thoroughly, trying to improve the suppleness of her spine. After treatment, she was again relaxed. I did mention her diet, but she did not respond.

Fourth visit

June reported that her back had felt 'much easier' during the last week. Her walk was not improved. The areas of redness remained. Her treatment continued as before, with emphasis on trying to increase the mobility of a very stiff spine.

Fifth visit

June talked in depth about her chronic back problems and the worry of having to take regular medication. We decided that, as she had received some pain relief from our sessions, she would continue to visit, but that she would also try to walk evenly on the soles of her feet. As she had been very upset, I massaged the solar plexus again, stimulating the adrenals; I worked on the spinal column and the cross-reflexes of her hip, and the knee was massaged. Her feet still smelt 'cheesy', so stimulation to the lymphatics was required to help toxin removal. After treatment, she was lively and relaxed and would visit in 2 weeks.

She continues to attend monthly for maintenance reflexology and pelvic girdle massage.

Mobility problems are commonplace in older adults and it appears that some may be amenable to complementary interventions. Caution must be exercised in any treatment so that longstanding conditions may be alleviated and not exacerbated.

Learning activity

1. To what extent is your care of these patients influenced by the medical model?
2. How would the integration of complementary therapies into your clinical area influence this?

References

Armstrong F (1991) Scenting relief. Nursing Times **87**(10): 52–53.

Arthritis News (1995) Special Edition: The balanced approach: a guide to drugs and complementary therapies. Arthritis News. Bristol: Audit Bureau of Circulations.

Arthritis Research Campaign (2000) Complementary Therapies and Arthritis. Information booklet. London: ARC.

Batehup L, Squires A (1992) Mobility. In: Redfern S (1992) Nursing Elderly People. Edinburgh: Churchill Livingstone.

Brown D (1993a) Headway Guides: Aromatherapy. London: Hodder & Stoughton.

Brown D (1993b) Headway Guides: Massage. London: Hodder & Stoughton.

Brownfield A (1998) Aromatherapy in arthritis. Nursing Standard **13**(5): 34–35.

Castell S (1999). Better balancing. Fitpro April/May: 25–27.

Cawthorne A (1991) Aromatherapy on trial. Aromanews **30**: 7–8.

Davis P (1999) Aromatherapy an A–Z, revised edn. Saffron Walden: CW Daniel Co. Ltd.

Department of Health (1998) Our Healthier Nation: A contract for health. London: HMSO Publications.

Howard J (1990) The Bach Flower Remedies Step by Step. Saffron Walden: CW Daniel Co. Ltd.

Johnson J, Pearson V, McDivitt L (1997) Stroke rehabilitation: assessing stroke survivors' long-term learning needs. Rehabilitation Nursing 22: 243–248.

Macdonald E (1995) Aromatherapy for the enhancement of the nursing care of elderly people suffering from arthritic pain. The Aromatherapist 2(1): 26–31 .

Marr J, Kershaw B (1998) Caring for Older People. London: Arnold.

Price S, Price L (1995) Aromatherapy for Health Professionals. Edinburgh: Churchill Livingstone.

Say B (1991) A panacea for all ills. Nursing Times 87(15): 58–60.

Simpson JM (1993) Elderly people at risk of falling: The role of muscle weakness. Physiotherapy 79: 831–835.

Stormer C (1995) Reflexology. The definitive guide. Reading: Hodder & Stoughton.

Tanner R (1990) Step by Step Reflexology. Surrey: Douglas Barry.

Vickers A (1996) Massage and Aromatherapy: A guide for health professionals. London: Chapman & Hall.

Vitti KA, Bayles CM, Crender WJ, Prendergast JM, D'Amico FJ (1993) A low-level strength training exercise program for frail elderly adults living in an extended attention facility. Aging 5: 363–369.

Watson S (1997) The effects of massage: an holistic approach. Nursing Standard 11(47): 45–47.

Williams MW, Nolan M (1993) Prevention of falls among older people at home. British Journal of Nursing 2: 609–613.

Williamson J, Smith RG, Burley LE (1987) Primary Care of the Elderly. Bristol: Wright.

Worwood V (1994) The Fragrant Pharmacy. London: Bantam Books.

CHAPTER 12

Sleeping and resting

Don't you know that four fifths of all our troubles in this life would disappear if we would just sit down and keep still.

Calvin Coolidge (30th President of the USA 1923–1929)

Sleep is essential to our well-being and yet it is often problematic. Indeed 10–15% of all adults who visit their general practitioner (GP) complain of chronic insomnia and it is the most frequently made health complaint (Mantle 1996). The physiology of sleep (Bouton 1986, Fox 1999), the problems associated with sleeping in hospital (Mantle 1996, Fox 1999, Arblaster and Carr 2000, Harvey 2000) and the difficulties associated with age-related changes in sleep patterns have all been well documented (Barnett et al. 1987, Kearnes 1989, Ersser and Taylor 1999). Barnett et al. (1987) identified how the need for sleep was reduced in old age to 5–7 hours, compared with a younger adult, who is said to need between 7 and 8 hours. Eliopoulos (1982) suggests that too much sleep may even be detrimental to an ageing individual because it may dull their senses. This is useful to know when assessing the sleep and rest requirements of older people.

It is essential, however, to acknowledge that, as this information is based on an average population, it needs to be interpreted with caution because each patient's needs are likely to deviate from any stated norm. Although older people might require less sleep, they will usually require more rest and it is thought that this time should be interspersed with some type of stimulating physical and mental activity throughout the day. Sleep and restlessness are therefore very subjective, personal experiences that are extremely hard to assess accurately.

One study (Ersser and Taylor 1999), which attempted to evaluate the effect of back massage on the sleep patterns of older people in care settings, was unable to identify this clearly because of the problems that they experienced when staff attempted to collect objective data about sleep patterns. Although the subjective data, amassed by the patients, proved very useful and easily accessible, the researchers noted how difficult it had been for nurses and carers to observe clearly and record exactly when patients went to sleep and also when they awoke.

Sleep has been defined as:

> ... a state of natural unconsciousness from which one can be aroused.
>
> Marieb (1995)

Bouton (1986) divided sleep into the following four stages:

Stage 1: falling asleep
Stage 2: slow wave sleep
Stage 3: rapid eye movement (REM) sleep
Stage 4: intermediate sleep

All stages follow a recognisable pattern but vary in length from individual to individual. Slow wave sleep is very light at first, but becomes deeper as it progresses. After this stage comes rapid eye movement (REM) sleep which is said to make up about 20% of an adult's sleep. Some people experience dreams or nightmares during this time. The final phase of REM sleep gives way to intermediate sleep, which prepares us for waking.

Others (Ornstein and Carstensen 1991) have described the sleep stages slightly differently, but recognise that the sleep cycle tends to be repeated several times and have suggested that REM sleep helps to restore the brain's mental processes whereas non-REM sleep helps restore the body (a greater explanation of this can be found in Bouton (1986) and Fox (1999)).

Older people report more sleeplessness than younger populations. Why do you think this is?
Identify factors that contribute to this and why.
What are the dangers of night sedation?

Sleeplessness is caused by the body not producing either enough of the sleep chemicals, particularly serotonin, or too much of the stimulating hormones such as adrenaline, cortisol and glucagon. In old age sleep is less deep and the deep sleep of stage 4 is said to be missing or greatly reduced. This reduction in the hours of REM sleep is, however, natural within this age group (Eliopoulos 1982, Mantle 1996) yet it often causes older people to think that they have a sleep problem when they are merely experiencing a natural reduction in sleep time. An older person, on waking, may also become very disoriented and even confused, and may need more time to adjust to this than someone who is younger. It is also sensible to allow them time to stretch and establish a good position before moving off!

Insomnia has many causes and it is the most common sleep disorder, taking many forms, including difficulties in: falling asleep, staying asleep and returning to sleep after waking prematurely, or, as seems to happen in many patients, a combination of all three (Mantle 1996) Although average sleep time decreases slightly with increased age, complaints of disturbed sleep appear to increase markedly as people get older and they often experience difficulty getting to sleep at night. Daytime napping and the nightly reliance on sedatives also compound the problem.

Mantle (1996) noted that the two major causes of insomnia within hospital settings appear to be directly related to the amount of pain or anxiety that a patient is experiencing. Out of the two, anxiety seems to be the most distressing symptom. Insomnia of course is therefore usually only a symptom secondary to a problem and Kearnes (1989) reported that maintenance of sleep was the most common form of insomnia in older people. She noted that the following problems impeded or disturbed an older person's sleep:

- Pain – from angina and migraine attacks, arthritic joints, peptic ulcer, leg cramps and gastro-oesophageal reflux.
- Dysuria, nocturia, with urinary bladder discomfort, incontinence and frequency of micturition.
- Constipation resulting from altered bowel habit or medication.
- Anxiety caused by being parted from a spouse, pet, or just his or her own home.

Unfortunately, as older people tend to experience chronic insomnia, they are often prescribed sedating drugs. The sleep-inducing drugs are classified as barbiturate and non-barbiturate and both may cause problems in old people. The former are rarely used nowadays because of their addictive nature and frequent use in the past as an aid to suicide. They should be used only with extreme caution because they depress many of the vital centres of the body. The *British National Formulary* (BNF 1999) states that before hypnotics are prescribed the cause of the insomnia should be established and, where possible, any underlying problems treated. As most sleep medication is effective only in the short term, it should be limited ideally to a maximum of 2 weeks!

Even excess non-barbiturate sedation may, because of its potential depression of the CNS, also create coordination problems and put older people more at risk of ataxia and falling and injuring themselves. The BNF (1999) advises that older patients should not be given hypnotics because of this and also that they exacerbate confusion, disorientation and even paradoxical and aggressive behaviour. This is particularly noted when benzodiazepines, such as nitrazepam and diazepam, are used as hypnotics. Long-term use of hypnotics may be counterproductive, because they often induce daytime sleepiness and sluggishness as well as night-time sleeping, as a result of the prolonged half-life of the medication.

How do you assess how much sleep or rest your patients are getting? Identify simple measures that could help patients to rest and sleep in your clinical area.

Simple measures can help occasional insomnia and these include the avoidance of: daytime napping or late morning sleeping and sleep-disturbing behaviour at bedtime, such as watching television and caffeine drinks. In addition to these, Rowlands (2000) also suggested that the following simple measures could be taken before going to sleep. She recommended that individuals should refrain from heavy meals, avoid sleeping pills and try to sleep in a well-ventilated, dark and quiet room. She also advocated some sort of relaxing activity such as meditation and/or a warm scented lavender bath. Although many authors have tended to concentrate purely on restricting caffeine, paying attention to diet and exercise to relieve chronic insomnia, Mantle (1996) believed that they were generally not sufficient on their own, but needed the added measures that Rowlands (2000) had listed. Mantle (1996) also favoured hypnosis and aromatherapy as sleeping aids.

It does appear that sleeping patterns can be learnt or re-learnt (Barnett et al. 1987). It is therefore important to look at ways in which patients may be helped to sleep and rest because sleep deprivation in hospital has been linked to diminished protein synthesis and immune function, and therefore thought to delay healing and recovery (Biley 1994, Topf et al. 1996).

Barnett et al. (1987) established that many factors affect an individual's sleep and things such as bedding, pillows and mattresses all contributed to poor sleep. The thing that appears to disturb sleep the most in institutions is, however, noise (Topf et al. 1996), and one small study (Arblaster and Carr 2000) sought ways to reduce this. The noises that they identified as being most troublesome were the unaccustomed ones such as staff chatting and walking in noisy shoes, beds being moved, call bells and machine alarms going off, doors opening and closing, and other patients snoring. This was compounded by late drug rounds and also lights being switched on and off during the night. Having identified these, they set standards to reduce them and after a 4-month period noted that most patient areas had demonstrated some improvement.

When helping patients to sleep, Fox (1999) states that it is very important to assess both their pre-sleep routine and those activities that are likely to settle them, and to record them in their care plan. She felt that patients' sleep routines could be helped and perhaps re-established by formulating individual sleep charts, which could record and evaluate the following:

- sleep habits
- sleep baselines
- pre-sleep routines
- interventions that may help an individual to sleep.

Which complementary approaches might help your older patients to sleep?

Therapeutic interventions

Having identified the sleeping difficulties and that medication is particularly troublesome in this age group, you need now to consider alternative interventions that may alleviate or reduce their problems. I find that as soon as this topic arises most people immediately think of aromatherapy and, in particular, oil of lavender. Perhaps this is because plant extracts have been used since time immemorial to aid health and well-being. Essential oils are, however, useful and as well as lavender there are many others that have the potential to induce sleep. Any of the sedating-type oils are suitable and these include Roman chamomile (*Anthemis nobilis*), neroli (*Citrus aurantium*), benzoin (*Styrax benzoin*), marjoram (*Origanum marjorana*) and clary sage (*Salvia sclarea*) (see Appendix I for further oils).

The essential oils do not work just by sedating the patient, but by treating any underlying problems that may be contributing to the insomnia, e.g. if the patient is very anxious, it may be useful to use neroli bigarade (*Citrus aurantium*) because it has been found to alleviate this anxiety, or if a patient has considerable arthritic joint pain, *Anthemis nobilis* (Roman chamomile), because of its anti-inflammatory properties, may reduce this. These can all be used very simply. Before going to bed, patients may enjoy a warm bath to which 6 drops of the chosen essential oil have been added, a hand or foot massage, or 2 drops could be put on to their pillow for them to inhale (or in a vaporiser).

Avis (1999) asserts that we need to think more about just how we use these essential oils. As a result of its name, she suggests that nurses tend to think that aromatherapy's method of application is by vaporisation. She warns that the indiscriminate use of scenting the patient environment is potentially dangerous and unethical because it may be 'unasked' for, and the appropriate informed consent may not have been obtained from all who might experience it. This will include, of course, not only patients but also relatives and staff alike! She said that to use essential oils responsibly must involve 'containing' that smell to the person who requires treatment (I was concerned about this in the case study later in the chapter). She also said that, when people are constantly bombarded with a smell, they get used to it and after a while are able only to sense larger amounts. She believes that it is therefore preferable to apply the essential oils to the skin in a diluted base oil so that the effect on others is reduced.

When reviewing the literature on sleep and complementary treatments, lavender does seem to be very influential and deserves a special mention. It has a wide range of therapeutic properties and there have been several studies, research based and otherwise, to support its use as a sedating agent. Passant (1990) observed how her older patients were more relaxed after she had used lavender (genus unspecified) with them. As she used it as part of a more holistic approach to care, however, it is difficult to establish to what extent the lavender may have contributed to this achievement.

When Buckle (1992) undertook a double-masked trial with massage using *Lavandula angustifolia* and *Lavandula bunatii*, she had some interesting results. Not only did she find that *L. bunatii* appeared to be twice as effective as *L. angustifolia* in relieving stress, after massage, but that there were three negative reactions to both oils recorded in the qualitative data.

Unfortunately, because of the inadequacy of the questionnaire, she was unable to identify whether it was the massage or the oils that they disliked!

Two further studies (Hardy 1991, Hudson 1996) used lavender as nocturnal sedation and, although the results were tenuous and as the populations studied were so small as not to be necessarily generalisable to other settings, they did indicate not only that their patients slept better but also that when they were awake during the day they were more alert and refreshed. Cannard's (1995) study also found not only that a commercially premixed blend of basil, juniper, lavender and sweet marjoram (genus not identified) helped most of his patients to sleep, but that the smell on the ward was very comforting.

Dunn et al. (1995) looked at the use of massage and aromatherapy, because of the widespread belief that they may offer intensive care patients more sensory input and some reduction in their stress and anxiety levels. As there is little objective evidence to support this, they designed a study to assess it. They randomly selected patients on admission to the intensive care unit (ICU) to have massage, aromatherapy and lavender oil or a period of rest. The data were gathered by objective testing and subjective patient evaluation questionnaires. Although the authors stressed that the results could not be generalised to other settings, of the three interventions those patients who received aromatherapy reported significantly greater improvements in their mood and perceived levels of anxiety. Although statistical results were not achieved, the patients' evaluations revealed that those who had received the lavender oil felt less anxious immediately after treatment, but the fact that they also felt more positive after treatment was not sustained.

Reflexology

A general reflexology treatment covering all of the reflexes will aid relaxation and overall calmness. Specific areas useful to treat are the head areas and those that are associated with any underlying problems that may inhibit or interrupt sleep, e.g. if a patient had indigestion it would be useful to treat the gut reflexes.

Bach and other flower remedies (see Chapter 5 for full list)

You could give Rescue Remedy to quiet an active mind and vervain (*Verbena officinalis*) is particularly useful to aid sleep in most patients. You can also use any of the remedies appropriately to combat the negative emotions that may be preventing sleep. An example of this would be giving a patient aspen if he or she is afraid but does not know why, or gorse if he or she is too despondent to sleep.

To what extent do you think you could use these interventions within your area of practice? What would stop you using them with your patients?

Combined treatments

Reflexology, aromatherapy and Bach flower remedies could be safely combined in one treatment, if you have the skills to do this. I have used, with one very anxious insomniac, a 5-minute hand reflexology treatment, the flower remedy vervain (*Verbena officinalis*) taken orally, in combination with the essential oil neroli bigarade (*Citrus aurantium*) added to the bath, with considerable success. Although neroli bigarade is one of the most expensive of the essential oils, I often use it, because it is very useful for combating anxiety and insomnia.

Breathing exercises, relaxation, imagery and other measures

Richards (1996) looked at other measures to aid sleep in older patients and tested the effect of a combination of muscle relaxation, mental imagery and relaxing music (MRMIM) and slow stroke back massage (SSBM) on the sleep and psychophysiological arousal of elderly men. The 69 men, all with a cardiovascular disorder, were randomly assigned, after admission to the critical care unit, to one of the two therapeutic groups or the control group. The control group received 'usual nursing care'. The results were encouraging. Although there were some significant differences in sleep time between the groups and patients accurately identified their own sleep times, the study also revealed that those who had experienced the two treatments had considerably less post-test anxiety than the control group. In addition, patients who had received the back rub felt better, more relaxed and could get off to sleep easier The study concluded that these interventions, which had focused on the body and mind connection, were potentially useful for promoting sleep in critically ill individuals.

It seems that regular periods of rest and relaxation are equally important to sleep for our physical and mental well-being, yet stress and anxiety often prevent us from benefiting from this. There are, however, very simple and effective measures that can be adopted to counteract their effects. Probably the most common measures are simple breathing exercises, which if practised regularly can ease tension, alter mental state and promote therapeutic relaxation. However, these practices are not new. Yoga and meditation have been practised by mystics for many thousands of years as a mental discipline to improve mental and physical health, and are now becoming valued in the West (Smith and Wilks 1997). For many centuries people have also believed in the power of prayer, and current evidence suggests that frequent personal prayer may help coping and psychological well-being (Maltby et al. 1999)

What do you think is involved in therapeutic relaxation?

Therapeutic relaxation involves more than just 'taking it easy' by listening to music or enjoying leisure pursuits. To be effective it needs to be a learnt and 'purposeful activity'. Fellows and Jones (1994) advise that to be competent in it will also require practice. Although there is no single definition of relaxation, all definitions appear to encompass the notion of excluding fear, anxiety and tension. There seem to be four main techniques.

What do you think the four main techniques are?

Muscle relaxation

This involves a progressive tensing and relaxing of the muscle groups, to achieve a relaxed state (Sims 1987). This is based on the idea that progressive muscle relaxation can undo the effects of stress and influence the state of the entire person. Relaxation techniques need to be simple enough so that people are able to follow easily and will also persevere with them

Visual guided imagery

Visualisation or guided imagery involves patients visualising themselves into different situations or settings to bring about any changes that they desire to make (Wills 1994). Although making images is a natural mental process, visualisation involves making a deliberate attempt to conjure up a positive picture in one's mind. Care must be taken when encouraging patients to do this, because visualisation is a very powerful force and may elicit images that are both unwanted and hard to dissipate. Used successfully, however, it can result in the ability to control and reduce tension, worry and anxiety and, if practised regularly, has the potential for self-healing and prevention of illness (Ryman 1994).

Meditative relaxation

This involves concentrating on an image, sound or phrase and ignoring everything else. It requires a passive attitude, quiet, comfortable positioning and repetition of the adopted phrase or word. It is suitable for all ages and does not rely on acceptance of any religious or philosophical belief. Therefore, as chanting is said to be helpful, during this activity patients may chant chosen words that are meaningful to them. Once comfortable with these words or phrase, it is said to be useful to keep using them during the entire relaxation period. Although it is suitable for all ages to pursue and has the potential to develop concentration, sensitivity and creativity, it is very difficult to achieve with patients in the short term because it requires a great deal of practice (Smith and Wilks 1997).

Breathing techniques

Diaphragmatic breathing can uniquely influence the unconscious processes of the body because, of all the functions directed by the autonomic (involuntary) nervous system, it is the easiest to control by will. Diaphragmatic, as opposed to chest, breathing will require practice and initially you may need to place one hand on the abdomen to see if the diaphragm and not just the chest muscles are moving. It is worthwhile pursuing because this slow rhythmical style of breathing facilitates relief of tension in the muscles. When discussing exactly how to breathe in this way, Leboyer (1985) advocated that in order to release this tension effectively, the 'secret' was to exhale slowly, using long and even breaths, so that the air was totally emptied from the both the lungs and the abdomen. This appears to be the exact opposite of what we have learnt to do, at this time, because normally during stressful situations the tendency is to hold your breath.

It appears that relaxation and visualisation could also work well together to provide a potential therapy that encourages positive and healthy rest and sleeping. The role of relaxation is to bring the mind to a state of balance and peace, and the use of relaxation techniques is becoming quite acceptable. Today a growing number of hospitals offer such therapies, on a regular basis, to both patients and staff (Ryman 1994). Within American hospitals, it is also quite common for patients to be taught some or a combination of them. They often also employ specialist practitioners who not only teach relaxation and visualisation techniques to the patients, but also educate them in supporting measures that might enable them to cope more effectively with their illnesses and perhaps enhance their own recovery (Goleman 1986). These therapies are either practised alone, as part of group therapy (with or without the support of a therapist), or by using audio-tapes, which combine music, imagery and relaxation techniques. Good (1995) noted that the use of audio-tapes is the best way of introducing these strategies into ward areas. Headsets may also reduce the sensory overload caused by increased noise and unfamiliar sounds, which O'Sullivan (1991) cites as being responsible for much of patient anxiety (see Chapter 10 for more on this).

I was inspired to try some of these approaches after I met an 'expert' relaxation nurse therapist, who worked in 'elder' care, at a 'Reflective Practice' conference in North Carolina. He detailed his experiences and gave practical demonstrations of how he used meditation, muscle tensing and breathing techniques, together with his older patients. Sometimes he left them with audio-tapes to reinforce his specific teaching. I was curious to see how this could work in some of the nursing home settings to which I have access.

To what extent do these theoretical perspectives on relaxation influence your current practice?

Evidence suggests that these initiatives could have an important part to play alongside conventional medicine because they have the potential for eliciting a state of physiological calm and a reduction in patient anxiety (Heidt 1991). Examples where these therapies have been used as effective nursing interventions include: the use of imagery within cancer care (Burke and Sikora 1992, Garnett 1994); as a therapy to ameliorate chronic and postoperative pain (McCaffrey 1990); for the 'natural' promotion of sleep instead of resorting to using sedating medication (Green 1994); for the alleviation of anger; and for patients recovering from myocardial infarction (Guzetta 1989).

O'Sullivan (1991) also notes that prolonged levels of anxiety and stress often cause an increase in sympathetic nervous system activity. This, in turn, may cause a rise in the levels of adrenaline and other cate-cholamines, which then leads to elevated heart rate and blood pressure, free fatty acid release, myocardial oxygen consumption, and a decrease in peripheral and renal perfusion. Then the risk of migrainal, hypertensive, cardiac, renal and cerebral disease all increases. Anxiety can also intensify muscle tension, which may exacerbate pain and serious postoperative complications. The systematic deep breathing employed when using relaxation and imagery is said to reduce postoperative pain by improving oxygenation levels and increased calmness. These alone help the patient cope with the trauma more easily, without resorting to large amounts of medication. As well as this, Green's (1994) review of the studies on deep relaxation showed improved lymphatic drainage, increased muscle flexibility and a correction of any pre-existing imbalance within the parasympathetic nervous system.

Cox and Hayes (1997) argued that nurses needed to employ these 'caring' skills alongside highly technological and procedural tasks, within hospitals, and I would suggest in other institutions, so that they can create a balanced environment that is more conducive to the reduction of anxiety and enhancement of patient comfort.

The following case study attempts to show how one elderly gentleman was helped to rest. Consider the implications for practice.

Alzheimer's disease: a case study

(First published in *Aromatherapy World* (1997) Distillation, pages 31–33; reproduced here by kind permission of the Editorial Board of the International Society of Professional Aromatherapists [ISPA]. The patient's name has been changed to ensure anonymity.)

Ron was referred to me by one of my post-registration students who worked in the nursing home where he was a patient. She wanted me to 'try' *Lavandula angustifolia* (lavender oil) to see if he could be helped to sleep or at least rest more. I was initially concerned about the legal and ethical implications of treating someone who was unable to give fully informed consent (Dimond 1995). Before assessing him I therefore sought permission from both the resident care manager and attending GP and, although they readily gave consent for me to proceed, I remained concerned about this even though several authors (Passant 1990, Hardy 1991, Buckle 1992) had suggested that touch and lavender (botanical name not always given) could help induce sleep in such patients.

Client background and presenting problems

This frail 94-year-old resident had been in care for 5 years. He was 165 cm (5 foot 6 inches) but only weighed just over 44 kg (7 stone). He neither smoked nor drank alcohol. He had suffered from rheumatoid arthritis for many years, which was well controlled by combined anti-inflammatory and analgesic drugs. Since 1989, however, he had suffered from Alzheimer's disease, which resulted in him going into care in 1992. The only other medication he was prescribed was night sedation – temazepam 5–10 mg at night.

When I visited the home, it was obvious that he was very difficult to care for. The staff thought that he needed a higher dose of night sedation because he was sleeping so little. The GP was reluctant to increase his medication because of the danger of inducing further confusion, even though the patient was very disruptive at night. Ron was also showing signs of short-term memory loss, which clearly manifested itself in the difficulties of remembering people and places.

Aim of treatment

To help Ron to sleep or at least be more restful.

Care plan

First treatment – initial assessment

I needed to build on the information already gained. Most of his relevant history was obtained from his carers. Neurologically, he displayed the classic signs of advanced Alzheimer's disease. He appeared anxious and very nervous, and had very little eye contact and no appropriate interactive skills. Loss of reasoning and thinking is more marked in the later stages of the disease (Cayton 1993).

He had no cardiovascular or respiratory problems and his skin, although paper thin over his shins, was very good for his age. He had some deformity present because of his arthritis, yet this did not affect his mobility. He had arthritic nodules on the fingers of both hands.

He was mostly incontinent of urine and faeces and underweight for his height, yet he remained well hydrated because he drank easily from a beaker. Although he was spoon-fed he still had difficulties in obtaining a proper diet because of his constant wandering and mental irritability.

Alzheimer's disease

Dementing illness is prevalent in 20% of those aged over 80 years. Of these it is thought that up to two-thirds have Alzheimer's disease (Alzheimer's Disease Society 1995). Although it is seen as a disease of old age, it has been estimated that there are 15 000 cases in the 40–60 age group (Cayton 1993). It is characterised by diseased or dead brain cells which cause progressive mental function deterioration. Although some research has suggested that altered genes (changing one of the brain's proteins) may be responsible, others have suggested that the disease is affected by aluminium or the presence of extra amyloid plaques in the brain (Redfern 1991, ADS 1995).

Current orthodox treatment centres on the identification of an accurate diagnosis and drug therapy. Neuropsychological approaches are increasingly being adopted because they are thought to give a greater insight into these patients' problems, especially in relation to their memory deficits. This is very pertinent for aromatherapists because there is evidence that such losses are associated with a damaged limbic system. Although a new cholinergic drug donepezil (Aricept), which works by slowing down the breakdown of acetylcholine – essential for brain nerve cell activity – and hopefully will help delay cognitive dysfunction for a while, has been licensed this year, it is thought to be associated with liver toxicity (Willis 1997). (Since writing this Aricept is now available for certain patients.)

First treatment – oils used and carrier

Alongside the above information, before treating Ron, I also considered the effects of both touch and essential oil toxicity on such a patient. As a result of his restless demeanour, it was difficult to communicate purposefully with him and, although it has been suggested that all patients benefit from touch, this is not necessarily so and it must be recognised that not all patients are receptive to touch (McCann and McKenna 1993). Although Horrigan (1995) stressed that massage could be startling or even cause further confusion in dementing patients, Miller (1995) felt that it could provide a meaningful communication tool.

In patients with Alzheimer's disease, who are robbed not only of their memory but also of their awareness, it is thought that scented oils may have the ability to act as a trigger and help them recapture some of their past experiences. Chrebet (1996) also feels that these oils could help in allaying anxieties and induce calmness without the utilisation of drastic medication regimens! Fowler and Wall (1997) urge caution when treating patients with aromatherapy in institutions. They argue that when using vaporised oils, people other than the chosen recipient of care will be affected, sometimes adversely. They stress that this is especially pertinent to consider where there are already people with cognitive impairment, such as the nursing home in which Ron resided.

As a result of this I chose to administer the essential oils only to him personally.

There is contradictory information surrounding the safety, toxicity and efficacy of essential oils, and much of the reasoning behind choosing any one oil, until recently, was often only anecdotal (Cawthorn 1995, Vickers 1996). Yet, more recently there have been a few published studies to inform practice and although Buckle's (1992) study was small she did find that *Lavandula angustifolia* (lavender) was more effective than *Lavandula bunatii* for reducing anxiety. Jager et al. (1992) also note its relaxing and sedating action. Although I could find no studies to support the use of *Anthemis nobilis* (Roman chamomile), not only had I been taught (Brown 1993) that it had anti-inflammatory and calming properties and that it had an affinity for dry and mature skin (for his arthritis), but in my own practice I had experienced this.

Consequently I mixed 1 drop each of *Lavandula angustifolia* and *Anthemis nobilis* in 10 ml of a composite carrier oil (he was not allergic to nuts, so I did not have to guard against this). I intended only to have superficial contact on this first visit, because I felt Ron was so confused that it would be best just to shake hands with him. I therefore applied the mix to my own hands and extended them to him. He readily took hold of them and while he continued to wander I carried on rhythmically stroking his hands and lower arms, talking to him gently at the same time. After approximately 10 min he became slightly agitated and restless, so I left him to wander on his own, under the watchful eye of a carer. I put 2 drops of *Lavandula angustifolia* on his pillow and also on a handkerchief that he had in his pocket. It was impossible to note if there had been any response.

Second visit – client response

I called in 2 days later to see him and when I introduced myself he did not remember me. There had been no improvement in his condition. I used the same mixture as before because I was concerned that he may be confused by differing aromas. I managed to massage both his hands and lower arms, and also to apply some gentle stroking movements to his forehead and scalp. He appeared really to like this. As before *Lavandula angustifolia* was dropped on to his pillow and handkerchief. In addition, I suggested that he was given some chamomile tea (see Hoffman 1960 for properties) before retiring. He continued with his night sedation.

Subsequent treatments

Third visit

I visited a week later in the late evening. He had not liked the chamomile tea so the nurse and I decided to try him with chamomile and apple tea instead. He was still very restless and not sleeping very well. We gently laid him on the bed and lifted his pyjama jacket and using the same mixture I managed to effleurage the whole of his back. He seemed soothed by this. With help I turned him over and firmly massaged both feet. I added *Lavandula angustifolia* and *Anthemis nobilis* (1 drop of each) to his pillow and handkerchief. He remained in bed. I left some of the mixture (4 drops of each per 30 ml) for the nurses to apply to his back and feet at bedtime.

Fourth visit

Ron was still wandering but the nurses thought he was slightly less distraught and more rested. I continued as before (visit 3) and left the same mixture. He had tolerated the tea.

Fifth visit (1 week later)

As above.

Sixth visit (1 week later)

Ron allowed a nurse and me to undress him and I massaged his back, paying particular attention to his pelvic girdle because of his arthritis; then as he remained still I attempted lymphatic drainage on both legs. He was less keen on this and hit out. To calm him we propped him face upwards and while I massaged his forehead and scalp the nurse gently stroked his hands. I again left the same mixture and applied the drops as before.

Seventh visit (1 week later)

The nurses reported that Ron had experienced one really restful night and although he was still wandering he was slightly less troublesome. Post-treatment instructions were as before.

Last visit (1 week later)

Ron continued to wander but appeared more at ease with himself. The nurses felt able to continue with his treatment themselves and were also considering whether they would use essential oils on other patients. I warned them of the dangers and implications of 'nurse dabbling' (Price and Price 1995, Tisserand and Balacs 1995), and they promised to consult with an aromatherapist before attempting this.

Results and reflections

It is difficult to show concrete and marked improvements in such a patient because of his poor mental and physical condition and prognosis. I was reluctant to overstimulate him or add any other oils because of the advice within current literature that says this may be detrimental to such patients (see 'Care plan'). As the nurses in the home wished to continue with his treatment and the referring nurse has left my course, I no longer have any dealings with the patient. I just hope that he may continue to feel at ease.

Having learnt that when using relaxation and other sleep and rest-inducing strategies it is essential to introduce them into quiet, uninterrupted and unhurried environments, I wondered just how hard this would be to achieve within busy institutions. It is obvious that before embarking on such initiatives it will be necessary to take extra measures to create this calm and private place. Simple things such as walking and talking quietly, pulling the screens around a bed, shutting a door and/or putting up 'Do not disturb' signs may be all that is needed!

References

Alzheimer's Disease Society (1995) Caring for Dementia. London: ADS.

Arblaster G, Carr S (2000) Silent night? Nursing Times **96** (41): 38–39.

Avis A (1999) When is an aromatherapist not an aromatherapist? Complementary Therapies in Nursing and Midwifery **7**: 116–118.

Barnett D, Knight G, Mabbott A (1987) Patients, problems and plans. Nursing Care of Patients with Medical Disorders. London: Edward Arnold.

Biley F (1994) Effects of noise in hospitals. British Journal of Nursing **3**: 110–113 .

BNF (1999) British National Formulary 38. London: British Medical Association and Royal Pharmaceutical Society of Great Britain.

Brown D (1993) Headway Lifeguides: Aromatherapy. Kent: Hodder & Stoughton.

Bouton J (1986) Falling asleep. Nursing Times December 10: 36–37.

Buckle J (1992) Which lavender oil? Nursing Times 88(22): 54–5.

Burke D, Sikora K (1992) Cancer: the dual approach. Nursing Times 88(38): 63–66.

Cannard G (1995) On the scent of a good night's sleep. Nursing Standard 9(34): 21.

Cawthorn A (1995) A review of the literature surrounding the research into aromatherapy. Complementary Therapies In Nursing and Midwifery 1: 118–120.

Cayton H (1993) Alzheimer's: Ageing painfully. Practice Nurse 1–13 July: 291–293.

Chrebet J (1996) Alternative Medicine. Aromatherapy and Alzheimer's. American Health Fitness of Body & Mind **15**(5): 29.

Cox L, Hayes J (1997) Reducing anxiety: the employment of therapeutic touch as a nursing intervention. Complementary Therapies in Nursing and Midwifery **3**: 163–167.

Dimond B (1995) Legal Issues – Complementary Therapies and the Nurse Complementary Therapies in Nursing and Midwifery **1**: 21–3.

Dunn C, Sleep J, Collett D (1995) Sensing an improvement: an experimental study to evaluate the use of aromatherapy, massage and periods of rest in an intensive care unit. Journal of Advanced Nursing **21**(1): 34–40.

Eliopoulos C (1982) Geriatric Nursing. London: Harper & Row Publishers.

Ersser S, Taylor H (1999) Measuring the sleep patterns of older people. Nursing Times **95**(1): 46–49.

Fellows B, Jones D (1994) Popular methods of relaxation: A survey with implications for therapy. Contemporary Hypnosis **11**: 99–109.

Fowler P, Wall M (1997) COSHH and CHIPS: ensuring the safety of aromatherapy. Complementary Therapies in Medicine **5**: 112–115.

Fox M (1999) The importance of sleep. Nursing Standard **13**(24): 44–47.

Garnett M (1994) Sounding it out. Nursing Times **90**(34): 64–68.

Goleman D (1986) Relaxation: surprising benefits detected. New York Times 13 May.

Good M (1995) Relaxation techniques for surgical patients. American Journal of Nursing **5**: 39–43.

Green L (1994) Touch and visualisation to facilitate a therapeutic relationship in an ITU: a personal experience. Intensive and Critical Care Nursing **10**(1): 51–57.

Guzetta C (1989) Effects of relaxation therapy on patients in a CCU with presumptive MI. Heart and Lung **18**: 609–616.

Hardy M (1991) Sweet scented dreams. International Journal of Aromatherapy **3**(1): 12–14.

Harvey A (2000) Pre-sleep cognitive activity: A comparison of sleep-onset insomniacs and good sleepers. British Journal of Clinical Psychology **39**: 275–286.

Heidt P (1991) Helping patients to rest: clinical studies in Therapeutic Touch. Holistic Nursing Practice **4**: 57–66.

Hoffman D (1960) The New Holistic Herbal. Shaftsbury: Element.

Horrigan C (1995) Massage. In: Rankin-Box D, ed., The Nurses' Handbook of Complementary Therapies. Edinburgh: Churchill Livingstone.

Hudson R (1996) The value of lavender for rest and activities in the elderly patient. Complementary Therapies in Medicine **4**: 52–57.

Jager W, Buckhaver, Jinoutz L, Fritzer M (1992) cited in Cawthorn (1995).

Kearnes S (1989) Insomnia in the elderly. Nursing Times **85**(47): 32–33.

Leboyer F (1985) The Art of Breathing. Dorset: Element Books Ltd.

McCaffrey M (1990) Nursing approaches to non. Pharmacological pain control. International Journal of Nursing Studies **27**(1): 1–5.

McCann K, McKenna H. (1993) An examination of touch between nurses and elderly patients in a continuing care setting in Northern Ireland. Journal of Advanced Nursing **18**: 838–846.

Maltby J, Lewis A, Day L (1999) Religious orientation and psychological well-being: The role of the frequency of personal prayer. British Journal of Health Psychology **4**: 363–378.

Mantle F (1996) Sleepless and unsettled. Nursing Times **92**(23): 46–47 .

Marieb (1995) Essentials of Human Anatomy and Physiology, 3rd edn. London: Benjamin Cumming .

Miller L (1995) The human face of elderly care. Complementary Therapies in Nursing and Midwifery **1**(4): 103–105.

Ornstein R, Carstensen T (1991) The Study of Human Experience, 3rd edn. New York: Harcourt Brace Jovanovich.

O'Sullivan R (1991) A musical road to recovery: Music in intensive care. Intensive Care Nursing 7: 160–163 .

Passant H (1990) An holistic approach in the ward. Nursing Times 86(4): 26–28.

Price S, Price L (1995) Aromatherapy for Health Professionals. Edinburgh: Churchill Livingstone.

Redfern S (1991) Nursing Elderly People, 2nd edn. Edinburgh: Churchill Livingstone.

Richards K (1996) Sleep promotion. Critical Care Nursing Clinics of North America 8(1): 39–52.

Rowlands B (2000) And so to bed ... but not to sleep. Candis January: 60–63.

Ryman L (1994) Relaxation and visualisation. In: Wells R, Tschudin V, eds, Wells' Supportive Therapies in Health Care. London: Baillière Tindall.

Sims S (1987) Relaxation training as a technique for helping patients cope with the experience of cancer: a selective review of the literature. Journal of Advanced Nursing 12: 583–591.

Smith E, Wilks N (1997) Meditation. London: Vermilion.

Tisserand R, Balacs T (1995) Essential Oil Safety. Edinburgh: Churchill Livingstone.

Topf M, Bookman, Arand D (1996) Effects of critical unit noise on the subjective quality of sleep. Journal of Advanced Nursing 24: 545–551.

Vickers A (1996) Massage and Aromatherapy: A guide for health professionals. London: Chapman & Hall.

Willis J (1997) The search for the key to Alzheimer's. Nursing Times 93(28): 40–41.

Wills P (1994) Visualisation. London: Hodder & Stoughton.

Further reading

Benson H, Klipper M (1997) The Relaxation Response. London: Collins.

Cook J (1986) Music as an intervention in the oncology setting. Cancer Nursing 9(1): 23–28.

CHAPTER 13

The cancer patient

The word 'cancer' and the term 'complementary medicine' have much in common because they are both generic names for diverse entities. The diagnosis of cancer still fills patients with horror and a variety of other emotions such as:

Rage, fear, confusion, a feeling of impotence and exile [are] all born out of that chilling word.

Graham (1983)

Cancer, from the Latin for crab, is the universal term for not just one disease but a broad spectrum of diseases with common features that may develop anywhere in the body. Cancer is a gene-based disorder, mediated by the activity of oncogenes and tumour suppressor cells and is caused by 'abnormalities in the mechanisms that control cellular growth and proliferation' (Morgan 2001). They are classified according to the type of tissue in which they are found, and their incidence is thought to be influenced by diet, lifestyle, smoking and the environment. The most common type of cancer is lung cancer, but for women breast cancer is the most commonly occurring (Morgan 2001).

Cancer can occur at any age and, although one in three people is likely to experience it, it will kill one in four of us (Department of Health 2000). As the incidence of most types of cancer increases with age, it is often seen as a disease of old age. Statistics reveal that more than 70% of all new cases occur in those over the age of 60 years (Cartmell and Reid 1993). Despite this very little is known about the biopsychological responses of older people to both cancer and the effects of its treatments, and there remains debate as to whether it is advancing age that increases cancer risk or whether it is more to do with people's prior health status (Given and Given 1989).

Despite some improvement and rationalisation in cancer management over the last few years, cancer remains the biggest single cause of death within the UK, killing 155 000 people per year. Although it is essential to remember that most will survive, many will not and it would seem that conventional methods of patient care do not always palliate or eliminate the effects of cancer either (White 1998). Although survival rates are strongly correlated to the standard of expert care available, services are often of varying quality, patchy and not equally available to all. In the European league tables, England and Scotland have both performed badly because their survival rates for the most common cancers lag behind most of Europe, they employ fewer oncologists per patient and spend less on anti-cancer drugs (Bower 1999).

As a result of this, various Government measures have been initiated to try to remedy some of these particular problems. In the NHS Cancer Plan (Department of Health 2000), the Government has pledged to invest an extra £570 million in cancer services by 2004. Its main aim is to save 10 000 lives by 2010 and it has also set the following targets, which must be achieved, at varying times, over the next decade:

1. Maximum wait times:
   - by 2001, patients should receive treatment for breast cancer within 1 month of diagnosis
   - by 2002, patients should receive treatment for breast cancer after urgent GP referral within 2 months
   - by 2005, all patients should receive treatment for all cancers within 1 month of diagnosis and within 2 months of urgent GP referral.
2. Breast screening should be also available to women aged 65–70 years by 2004.
3. Smoking should be reduced from the 1998 levels of 32%, in manual workers, to 26% by 2010.

Centres that do not achieve these targets may have their services withdrawn and transferred elsewhere. In addition to this, the NHS Executive (2000) initiative has given nurses a major role to help achieve these. Nurses are to have more educational opportunities, be encouraged to develop more specialist roles and have extra nursing research funded. There are already fears, however, that the current nurse shortages and, in particular, the low numbers of specialist cancer nurses will erode many of these opportunities (Ward and Wood 1999).

Much of the above addresses issues relating to cure, but often does not consider how patients will cope with this disease. Complementary therapies appear to have a substantial and increasing part to play (White 1998). The most common therapies that are used by nurses with cancer patients seem to be massage, aromatherapy, reflexology, and, more recently, flower remedies and acupuncture and acupressure. They do not claim to cure, but are useful as an adjunct to orthodox care, and it seems that patients request complementary therapies mostly for stress relief and to help their musculoskeletal problems (Downer et al. 1994).

There is a vast amount of literature amassing on the complementary care of cancer patients, very little of which pertains exclusively to older people and much of it is purely anecdotal. Within this literature, I found only one, American, survey that looked particularly at older people and their use of complementary therapies, while receiving conventional medical treatments. This study recruited 699 patients aged over 69 years, from community cancer centres, in the State of Michigan. The results, gained from patient self-report data, showed that approximately 33% of them were using complementary therapies, the most frequent of which were herbal therapies and spiritual healing. The users were more likely to be better-educated women diagnosed with breast cancer. All users were, however, deemed to be more optimistic about their future and had experienced significantly more improvements in their physical symptoms than non-users (Wyatt et al. 1999).

There have also been several other surveys and evaluative studies that have looked at both the efficacy of treatments and why people might be accessing them. Studies, such as those of Slade (1992) and Downer et al. (1994), have noted that cancer patients often accessed and chose to use such therapies alongside their conventional treatments, and that increasingly specialist centres were providing them. Although there is evidence of increased usage, White (1998) observed that it was very difficult to identify what that actually meant, because the questionnaire used did not allow for greater clarification, e.g. when managers at the centres replied that they were using aromatherapy, it was impossible to differentiate between the use of essential oils within a prescribed massage programme directly with patients or when oils were merely 'burnt' to scent patient areas.

It is of interest that the study of Downer et al. (1994) revealed that, even when complementary therapies had little impact on their illness, patients were still satisfied with their chosen therapies. The only dissatisfaction that they reported was in relation to the awful side effects of conventional therapies and the fact that such practitioners gave them no hope for the future (more will be said in Chapter 15 about this).

Turton and Cooke (2000) were amazed how little attention focused on what patients actually wanted from the therapies themselves. They added that, even today, health professionals make most of the decisions unilaterally, and predominantly unchallenged, about the care that an individual patient will be given. As a result of this, their study, using focus groups, sought to elicit specific information from patients and their carers about their needs during the 'cancer journey'. Their findings were complex because they encompassed information from four key areas:

1. The emotional cancer journey. Here patients identified a whole range of emotions ranging from shock and disbelief to feelings of 'why me', which they experienced after being diagnosed with cancer.
2. Self-management strategies and sources of support. As part of their own self-management process, many of the study participants revealed that using complementary therapies was an important part of this. They used them because it made them feel empowered, individual and in control, and also that it helped their symptom management by more 'natural' means.
3. The medical interface. Here patients stressed that, as the initial contact between them and health professionals was so crucial, they urged that this should be conducted sympathetically and also that a greater understanding of the importance of self-management should be shown.
4. Carers and relatives. This revealed that carers were often overprotective of their loved ones, but also felt marginalised by professionals because they were allowed very little input into any care decisions.

From this study the following recommendations were made:

1. The medical interface should be improved to take more account of the patients' psychological state and to adopt supportive practices which will allow patients to retain much of the control over their own health.
2. Appropriate support services should be set up, including access to a broad range of self-help and treatment options.
3. Policies should be actively developed to ensure the above.

This is very much the supporting philosophy of the Bristol Cancer Centre (Turton and Cooke 2000) and probably many of the others.

Self-help and charitable initiatives

There are many charitable and voluntary organisations around the country that seek to support patients with complementary therapies. The Bristol Cancer Centre pioneered much of this work, and others such as the Haven Trust (Davenport 1998) and the Cancer Resource Centre (Carlowe 2000) have followed. The latter two centres were both created by members of the general public who had suffered bad experiences within orthodox care. Not only do such centres offer a chance for patients to experience a range of tactile therapies, but they also allow patients to express their feelings freely about their diagnosis and prognosis. It has been suggested that such places encourage patient self-empowerment and realistic hope (see Chapter 14).

Locus of control and placebo effect

Complementary therapies therefore have the potential not only to help patients cope with the inherent anxiety and stresses of their illness but also often to provide effective symptomatic relief as well. At the terminal end of cancer care they can also help the grieving processes associated with loss and bereavement. As one in three patients will be affected by cancer, there is an urgent need for us to develop more holistic and patient-centred models of care (Burke and Sikora 1992). This is especially relevant when one thinks of the many traumatic and distressing orthodox interventions that patients may have to suffer and although patients such as Izod (1996), when writing about his personal cancer journey, stated that whilst he recognised that his survival was a result of the high technology of modern oncology treatments, they had not helped him to cope with the resulting psychological distress, boredom or dreadful experiences. Instead he had relied on a friend who 'rubbed [his] scalp in a soothing fashion'. Not only did this help him to cope with his therapy, but it also assisted him in coming to terms with his diagnosis and made him more open to 'self-healing'. He added that:

> I can see no problem in promoting complementary therapies on the grounds that they are simply nice, and having nice things done to my body when everybody else was either sticking needles in it, cutting it open or trying to poison it, is surely going to have some beneficial effects. I really don't think that one need make any greater claim than that, for that is surely enough!
>
> Izod (1996)

Over the last few years there has been more interest in the use of aromatherapy massage for cancer patients as an adjunct to medical treatment. Although more nurses are using aromatherapy massage, there is little research to illustrate its effectiveness in patient care. One study (Wilkinson 1995) was set up not only to evaluate the effectiveness of massage and aromatherapy massage in improving the quality of life for patients with advanced cancer, but also to find out about whether patients perceived that aromatherapy massage helped to improve quality of life. Fifty-one day patients or inpatients, who attended the Liverpool Marie Curie Centre and had been referred for massage, were invited to participate in the study. They were selected for either a full aromatherapy body massage with Roman chamomile, diluted in a base oil, or a full body massage using only a carrier oil. They all received three full massages over a 3-week period.

Each patient was tested before and after the massage, using an established symptom checklist and the Spielberger Trait Anxiety Inventory. Two weeks after their last massage, they were encouraged to complete a questionnaire. The data were analysed using non-parametric statistical tests and the results demonstrated improved post-test scores for both the massage and aromatherapy massage patients. As the patients perceived massage and aromatherapy massage to be very helpful for reducing tension and anxiety and also for pain relief, the study concluded that aromatherapy massage may have a role to play in improving the quality of life of advanced cancer sufferers.

To date, there is very little research into the use of reflexology with cancer patients and one, recent, very small-scale study (Hodgson 2000) sought to remedy this. The study's aims were to find out what the perceived effects of reflexology were, whether it impacted on patients' quality of life and also if such a service should be provided, within a general setting, for palliative care. Only 12 patients in the palliative stage of their illness, who were aware of their diagnosis and had never previously experienced reflexology, were attracted to the study. These patients were randomly assigned to a reflexology or placebo group and before and within 24 hours of completion of the treatment the participants were asked to complete a visual analogue scale (VAS).

The results were interesting, although, on her own admission, they may have been flawed, because as a result of a typing error the author failed to use five of the borrowed VAS components. All 12 patients reported enjoyment of the experience; however, only two of the placebo (control) group, as opposed to all six of the reflexology group, noted any benefit in their quality of life. Although advising caution and also recognising that these results were not necessarily generalisable to other cancer populations, the researcher did feel that her study suggested some improvement in her patients' quality of life and many of their symptoms, and that there was a place for this provision within a hospital setting.

Myths and misunderstandings

There are some very common myths and fears associated with the use of complementary approaches in cancer care, especially in relation to the use of massage and essential oils. As Kassab and Stevensen (1996) state, all too often this misinformation arises out of hearsay evidence and pure conjecture. Possibly the most common myth is the assertion that massage spreads cancer by stimulating the lymphatic circulation. As the stimulation to this system during massage is no more than that experienced during everyday activities, it seems that cancerous spread is just as likely to occur by natural rather than by other means. Tisserand and Balacs (1995) note that there is no scientific evidence to support or disprove this. Although opinions on this vary, most people feel that it is best to avoid any deep tissue massage, especially over the tumour site and surrounding lymph glands, and as irradiated skin is very friable it should not be massaged either.

Concerns have also been expressed about using reflexology and other zonal therapies with cancer patients. Kassab and Stevensen (1996) believe that these have arisen because of unfounded fears of metastatic spread and enhanced excretory action. They also state that there is no evidence to support even the view that patients receiving cancer drugs will not benefit, because the drugs after reflexology will be 'hurried' through the system. As such drugs normally have a half-life, it is unlikely that gentle foot massage will affect them.

Another misconception is that many of the essential oils are capable of actually inducing cancer, but Tisserand and Balacs (1995) argue that there is no evidence to support this. Although, undoubtedly, there are a few essential oils that contain potentially carcinogenic substances, they are known and need not be used.

As a result of these issues, guidelines have been produced by some of the therapy organisations for their individual members' use and also by the Royal College of Nursing, for those working with aromatherapy within care settings. This latter document, published last year in the *Complementary Therapies Nursing Forum Newsletter* (Anon 2000) advised the following.

Guidelines

1. Written medical consent must be obtained before treatment. The following categories of patients should not be treated: (a) any patient for 6 months after surgery, radiation or chemotherapy; (b) patients with petechiae, excessive bruising or a platelet count lower than $80 \times 10^9/l$; or (c) patients with unresolved symptoms, unless express medical permission allows this. Stringer (2000) noted how the leukaemic patients on her unit were 'walking contradictions to massage', because they had no white cells or platelets and were very susceptible to rashes and infections, some of which were drug induced. Yet initial evaluation of her massage programme reveals that the massage had relaxed and soothed the patients as well as easing much of their physical pain.
2. The therapist must be adequately and appropriately trained in both aromatherapy and cancer care, and should initially be supervised in this practice. They should also have access to the book by Tisserand and Balacs (1995) on essential oil safety.
3. Massage should consist of light effleurage strokes only and lymphoedema massage (see Chapter 3) should not be attempted unless the therapist is also qualified in this additional technique.
4. Aromatherapy should be avoided if there are any skin imperfections, wounds, rashes, etc., and essential oils should not be applied directly to any open or fungating wounds.
5. The essential oil concentration should only be 1%, e.g. to each 5 ml of carrier oil, only 1 drop of essential oil should be added. Although this document does not specify dosage when patients are also having ortho-dox cancer treatment, it is likely that the dilution would need to be even lower (Cawthorne and Carter 2000). Any side effects must be reported.

Cawthorne and Carter (2000) state that aromatherapy and massage both need to be modified when dealing with cancer and palliative care patients. They advise that massage should avoid the primary tumour site, any enlarged lymph nodes, and thrombosed and lymphoedematous limbs. In addition to this, they have devised a modified aromatherapy or massage technique and called it the HEARTS process. This mnemonic stands for:

Holding – this relates to the touch that is given during massage and they feel that this is vitally important because it can convey love to patients at such a vulnerable time in their lives.

Empathy – this encompasses touch, relaxing music and verbal and non-verbal communication between the patient and therapist so that the therapist may be 'in tune' with the patient's needs.

Aromatherapy – this involves the choice of appropriate oils to promote relaxation and reduce anxiety.

Relaxation – here music and verbal skills are used to promote a relaxation response.

Therapeutic relationship – the authors note that this is the most important aspect of this process because when mutual trust is built up therapy is likely to be more effective.

Stroking – light strokes are applied using the hands or fingers only and this can either be applied directly to the skin or through a cover depending on the needs of the individual patient.

This does seem to be a very useful philosophy of care to adopt.

Practical suggestions for treatment
(many of these will also be applicable to use within Chapter 14)

Only safe and practical measures such as the cautious use of aromatherapy blends, massage, reflexology, flower remedies and relaxation are included. Patients with cancer will present with very many different symptoms, and be at very different stages and degrees of severity of their treatments and length of their personal cancer journey. Please note, therefore, that these are all very general examples, the use of which will depend on the individual needs of your patients, their condition, their prescribed current orthodox treatment and also the contraindications for practice. I have found them to be useful, however. As a result of the individuality of the patient, some modification may have to be made. Remember only those who are appropriately competent and permitted to do so should practise them. In addition to this, there are a few essential oils that are best avoided. In the absence of conclusive evidence and, although there is debate between different authors on this, in the main they include those listed below.

Essential oils to avoid

- *Ocimum basilicum* (basil) because it is feared that it is carcinogenic and hepatoxic, especially if the estrazole is more than 10%.
- *Cinnamum zelanicum* (cinnamon) because it inhibits blood clotting and may be hepatoxic.
- *Syzgium aromaticum* (clove) has a similar action to cinnamon but is also thought to inhibit platelet activity.
- *Foeniculum vulgare* (fennel) is deemed to be potentially carcinogenic.

- *Achillaea milliefolium* (yarrow), *Hyssopus officinalis* (hyssop), *Rosemarinus officinalis* (rosemary) *Salvia officinalis* (sage – Dalmation), *Salvia lavandula* (sage – Spanish) are all said to be neurotoxic.
- *Litsea citriadora* (verbena) is a known dermal irritant and may also increase dermal sensitivity and phototoxicity

Further information about essential oils not listed in Appendix I can be found in Brown (1993), Davis (1999), and Price and Price (1995).

Coping with altered body image

Many of the problems listed below are associated with patients' perceptions of their visible or invisible altered body image. This is an intensely personal experience and, although it will not affect all patients, it can often impinge on an individual's quality of life (see Chapter 14). As it is so personally defined, successful coping will be very individual and depend on not only the value systems of patients, but also how they are helped to adjust to any alteration (Price 1990). Bound up with all of this are huge physical and emotional components that influence very much how we see ourselves and how we want others to see us. It is essential that carers recognise this because any disapproval from others at this time could cause extra stress.

Price (1990) noted that body image is a very complex, constantly changing notion, bound up with sexuality (which may also be gender specific), culture and age. He argued that it is made up of five separate components:

1. Body reality (as it really is) influenced by ageing, fitness, physical abilities and control of these, and sensory faculties.
2. Body ideal (as we would like it) influenced by social, peer, cultural and own norms, fashion, advertising and own coordination.
3. Body presentation influenced by wealth, aesthetics, appendages (stick), environment.

He asserts that we try daily to balance these and are in turn influenced by:

4. Coping strategies, such as subconscious (grief) rationalisation and social conformity plus our own.
5. Social networks, which may be extensive or otherwise, responsive or not, clear or confused, geographically varied, and either ignorant or insightful about body image concerns.

The key to understanding how others feel about their body image is to try to comprehend the patients' own value systems, especially in relation to their own body image and how they cope with any deviations from the norm. Altered body image does not therefore concern only the visibly obvious, such as the amputation of a limb or a breast (mastectomy), stoma formation, and other maiming features such as hair loss, but also less visible changes such as impotence and frigidity, especially if the prognosis is poor. As self-image and self-esteem are so interconnected, it may be that patients will be helped to come to terms with any change if their physical appearance can be enhanced in any way. This not only includes how they look but also how they smell (see below)!

- Pain is often one of the most feared consequences of cancer and its treatments and is said to distort body image, because any poorly controlled pain tends to dominate the patient's total thoughts. Massage, relaxation (see Chapters 12 and 14), many of the essential oils and reflexology have a part to play in this management of pain. Pain often has varying components so it is sensible to blend oils that include analgesic properties such as *Mentha piperita* (peppermint), *Lavandula angustifolia* (lavender), *Zingiber officinale* (ginger) with *Anthemis nobilis* (Roman chamomile) because of its anti-inflammatory properties. Pain also has an emotional component and oils that are suitable for this are anxiolytics such as *Citrus aurantium* (neroli bigarade) and others such as *Rosa damascena* (rose), *Citrus bergamia* (bergamot), *Santalum album* (sandalwood) or *Pelargonium odorantissimum* (geranium). By managing pain effectively many of the other symptoms such as fatigue and sleeplessness often disappear.
- Muscle tension may be relieved by massage, with or without relaxing oils such as *Boswellia thurifera* (frankincense), *Pelargonium odorantissimum*, *Lavandula angustifolia* and *Citrus aurantium*.
- Constipation and diarrhoea are very common problems within cancer care. Stringer (2000) felt that cancer patients often got 'sucked' into a vicious cycle of drug dependency and the associated problems of drug interaction. She gave an example of the 'upset bowel', which she believed was an iatrogenically induced problem because patients, after they have routinely been given treatments that either constipate or cause them to have diarrhoea, have to have either of these conditions reversed by yet another drug. She felt that it might be better to relieve these symptoms by gentle abdominal massage, instead of

relying on even more drugs (see Chapter 9 for this and other examples of symptomatic relief).

- Nausea: anti-nausea oils include *Mentha piperita*, *Lavandula angustifolia* and *Zingiber officinale*.
- Breathing difficulties: useful oils to help alleviate breathing and congestive difficulties include: *Mentha piperita*, *Lavandula angustifolia*, *Melaleuca leucadendron* (cajuput) (more are listed in Chapter 8).
- Recurrent infections and wound care: although fungating wounds are relatively uncommon, and as healing is very unlikely, their care is often problematic. Often such wounds ulcerate into the surrounding tissues and smell very offensive. It is this smell that is often the most distressing symptom for individual patients. These wounds are very hard to treat and, as it is not recommended to apply oils directly to such areas, it may be that treatment will concentrate on helping disguise the smell and assist any other symptoms. The choice of a sweet smelling oil is probably best left to the individual patient to decide. But oils such as rose, jasmine, lavender and the citrus oils are all suitable.
- Mood fluctuations are often present and may be helped by the use of uplifting oils such as *Boswellia thurifera*, *Citrus bergamia*, *Citrus aurantium*, *Santalum album* and *Rosa damascena*, for balancing the psyche. Soothing oils include *Lavandula angustifolia* and *Citrus aurantium*, and *Vetiveria zizanoides* (vetivert) and *Jasminum officinale* (jasmine) are both especially useful when grieving and/or crying.
- Fatigue can be an all-embracing affliction emanating from both the cancer and its treatment outcomes. Patients need to be advised to rest, and to consider their diet options and lifestyle. Oils such as *Melaleuca alternifolia* (tea tree), *Citrus limonum* (lemon) and *Lavandula angustifolia* are all said to strengthen the immune response. Massage with a combination of them may help. Patients, perhaps also because of pain or anxiety, experience insomnia and/or disturbed sleep. Chapter 12 gives a comprehensive assessment of this. Terminal restlessness may be alleviated by *Santalum album* and *Rosa damascena*.
- Associated surgical, radiotherapy and chemotherapy treatments: for varying reasons caution will need to be exerted here. For patients undergoing chemotherapy, it is essential not to use anything on them that may compete for the binding sites on the plasma albumin (Miller 1996). Once it was thought that these patients should not receive aromatherapy at this time, but Price and Price (1995) advise that, with care, patients may benefit from specific area massage. As cytotoxic drugs affect the haemopoietic system, these patients may suffer from

anaemia, lethargy and pallor, and may also suffer from bleeding gums, increasing fatigue and dyspnoea.

More than 40% of cancer patients undergo radiotherapy (Miller 1996). Usually the treatment is localised and marked accordingly. Side effects tend to include anorexia, nausea, vomiting and fatigue, caused by the release of metabolites into the systemic circulation during the breakdown of the tumour during treatment. As the site of irradiation must be avoided, any massage or use of oils must be applied to other areas of the body. Increasingly, evidence suggested that skin prepared with essential oils, such as *Melaleuca alternifolia* and *Anthemis nobilis*, 3 weeks before treatment will prevent or decrease burning and scarring (Miller 1996).

Before and after surgery, patients may enjoy a familiar scent added to the environment and may benefit from a massage or aromatherapy massage, using oils suitable for their condition, away from the site of the surgical incision

The oils should therefore be chosen to ameliorate any side effects, raise self-esteem and boost the immune system. By selective blending, two or three oils may be combined to make an appropriate synergistic blend (see Appendix I and Chapter 5).

Reflexology

Using lighter pressure, if necessary, a complete reflexology treatment is likely to benefit these patients because of the relaxing effects that it produces, but will depend on their stage of treatment and severity of illness. If patients are not well enough for this, it is useful to pay attention to the zones affected, and treat either the disease and/or symptom-specific area. It is very useful to treat both of the solar plexus and the adrenal areas, because they are helpful for allaying anxiety and inducing calmness. Never over-stimulate at this time.

Flower remedies

Many of the flower remedies could be used for patients and their carers during this time and it may be useful if you consult the full list presented in Chapter 6. I would particularly recommend those used to remedy: apprehension and fear, such as mimulus and/or aspen; despondency, despair and exhaustion, especially gorse, crab apple and star of Bethlehem; uncertainty, for patients, but especially carers, scleranthus or wild oat; and also the composite Rescue Remedy for anguish, panic, shock and other emergency situations.

Hospice care

Within hospice care, 'bought in' services or volunteers still primarily provide complementary therapies, although there is evidence that nurses are now increasingly involved in their provision as part of in- and outpatient care (White 1998). The therapies are used in a variety of ways but often this entails providing emotional support for both the dying patient and their formal and informal carers, aiding purposeful relaxation and the alleviation of generalised symptomatology.

Alternative treatments/cures

Lastly it is essential for you to be aware of competing alternative therapies, which patients may want to access. Although there is increasingly more information about how cancer patients combine both orthodox and complementary treatments, there is very little available to inform us why people choose not to continue with orthodox oncology and seek another alternative treatment. One small investigation (Montbriand 1997) felt that some of this might be because minimal attention has been given to this subject. This ethnographic study, however, after exploring abandonment theories, concluded that anger seemed to precipitate this event. By abandoning the conventional for the alternative, their hopes for a cure seemed to be raised 'to the extremes of illusion and denial of possible death'. It was also suggested that this study could raise orthodox practitioners' awareness and possibly help them avoid the problem in the beginning, or at least facilitate estranged patients' return to medical care.

Undoubtedly, there are some unusual and, to traditionalists, somewhat alarming therapies and 'cures' offered in the name of alternative therapy. Kassab and Stevensen (1996) stated that the problem with many alternative treatments was that they were marketed as cures and yet there was no evidence to support this. Bell and Sikora (1996) and Kassab and Stevensen (1996) both list a few of the treatments with names such as essiac, laetrile, shark's cartilage, rebirthing, radionics, Gerson and Livingstone therapies, the use of Shitakii mushrooms and Hoxsey, to name but a few! I must admit to never having heard of many of them and I have also been unable to find anything about some of them within the literature. It would therefore be very difficult for me to comment on them but, like Bell and Sikora (1996), I would expect them to be subject to the same scrutiny as other therapies. Of course patients are able to exercise their own choice about treatments, although it may be preferable if the choices they make are informed!

The word 'cancer' still evokes terror in the hearts of many of us and this appears to be exacerbated when considering using complementary therapies. There are still many myths and taboos, often born out of the hearsay and conjecture that surround and ultimately influence their use. This is tragic because, although not claiming to cure, undoubtedly they do have a major and increasing role to play in the care of people with cancer. Their introduction into care is often not influenced by healthcare professionals, but at the behest of patients themselves. It would seem that, as professionals, we need to recognise this and be more proactive in our practices, because, used appropriately, they have the potential to help patients live through their cancer journey, to either recovery or death.

Learning activity

Imagine that you are about to set up a complementary therapy service for cancer patients within your area of practice. Using the following questions to guide you, devise a realistic and cost-effective action plan. This needs to be supported by a clear rationale and an implementation strategy. Before doing this, you need to think clearly about the implications of this for both you and the patients involved. To help you with this task, you will need to refer to other chapters in the book and perhaps also discuss some of the arising issues with others in your area.

1. What complementary therapies are available and which ones are most suitable to use?
2. Who is competent to practise them and how may you assess this? Will you consider 'buying' in the services of a non-nurse therapist? If you do are there other contractual and professional issues to consider?
3. What are the implications for using massage, aromatherapy, reflexology and flower remedies with cancer patients? What are the specific contradictions to using them?
4. Are there any national and local guidelines to abide by? What are the legal, ethical, political managerial and professional influences that may impinge on their safe introduction?
5. Who will fund them, because they cannot be provided at the expense of orthodox therapies? Is it possible to treat all cancer patients in this way, are they suitable to use with the newly diagnosed and/or acutely

ill patients or would it be better just to use them on chronically sick patients?

6. If your complementary service becomes very successful and patients decide that they will not use their conventional medication, etc. anymore, how will you deal with this? If patients are keen to know about and possibly use an alternative to orthodox treatments, such as *Iscador* (mistletoe), shark's cartilage or psychic surgery, how will you advise them?

7. Who will benefit the most from this activity?

I have suggested that you contemplate the above task because it contains many of the elements that you are likely to encounter when attempting to introduce therapies into any area of orthodox practice. Good luck!

References

Anon (2000) Aromatherapy guidelines for treating people with cancer. In Touch. London: Royal College of Nursing.

Bell L, Sikora K (1996) Complementary therapies and cancer care. Complementary Therapies in Nursing and Midwifery 2: 57–58.

Bower H (1999) Own goal in the European league. Nursing Times 95(20): 26–27.

Brown D (1993) Headway Guides: Aromatherapy. London: Hodder & Stoughton.

Burke C, Sikora K (1992) Cancer – the dual approach. Nursing Times 88(38): 62–66.

Carlowe J (2000) The comfort zone. Nursing Standard 14(39): 14–15.

Cartmell B, Reid M (1993) Cancer control and epidemiology. In: Groenwald S et al., eds, Cancer Nursing Principles and Practice, 3rd edn. London: Jones & Bartlett.

Cawthorne A, Carter A (2000) Aromatherapy and its application in cancer and palliative care. Complementary Therapies in Nursing and Midwifery 6: 83–86.

Davenport S (1998) The Haven Trust Newsletter Issue 1.

Davis P (1999) Aromatherapy an A–Z, revised edn. Saffron Walden: CW Daniel Co. Ltd.

Department of Health (2000) NHS Cancer Plan: A plan for investment, a plan for reform. London: The Stationery Office.

Downer S, Cody M, McClusky P et al. (1994) Pursuit and practice of complementary therapies by cancer patients receiving complementary therapies alongside conventional treatment. British Medical Journal 309: 86–89.

Given B, Given W (1989) Cancer nursing for the elderly: a target for research. Cancer Nursing 12(2): 71–77.

Graham J (1983) In the Company of Others – Understanding the Human Needs of Cancer Patients. Suffolk: St Edmundsbury Press.

Hodgson H (2000) Does reflexology impact on cancer patients' quality of life? Nursing Standard 14(31): 33–38.

Izod D (1996) A patient's perspective. Complementary Therapies in Nursing and Midwifery 2: 66–67.

Kassab S, Stevensen C (1996) Common misunderstandings about complementary therapies for patients with cancer. Complementary Therapies in Nursing and Midwifery 2: 62–65.

Miller R (1996) The use of aromatherapy in hospitals for patients with cancer. The Aromatherapist 3(2): 14–29.

Montbriand M (1997) The 1996 Schering Lecture: An inquiry into the experience of oncology patients who leave biomedicine to use alternative therapies. Cancer Oncology Nursing Journal 7: 6–13.

Morgan C (2001) Making sense of cancer. Nursing Standard 15(20): 49–53.

NHS Executive (2000) The Nursing Contribution to Cancer Care. London: Department of Health.

Price B (1990) Body Image: Nursing concepts and care. London: Prentice Hall.

Price S, Price L (1995) Aromatherapy for Health Professionals. Edinburgh: Churchill Livingstone.

Slade S (1992) Alternative/complementary medicine in radiotherapy. Radiography Today 58: 13–16.

Stringer J (2000) Massage and aromatherapy on a leukaemia unit. Complementary Therapies in Nursing and Midwifery 6: 72–76.

Tisserand R, Balacs T (1995) Essential Oil Safety: A guide for health care professionals. Edinburgh: Churchill Livingstone.

Turton P, Cooke H (2000) Meeting the needs of people with cancer for support and self-management. Complementary Therapies in Nursing and Midwifery 6: 130–137.

Ward J, Wood C (1999) Cancer care: how nurses cope. Nursing Times 95(49): 50–51.

White P (1998) Complementary medicine a treatment of cancer: a survey of provision. Complementary Therapies in Medicine 6: 10–13.

Wilkinson S (1995) Does aromatherapy enhance the quality of life of patients with advanced cancer. Psycho-Oncology 4: 98.

Wyatt G, Friedman L, Given C, Given B, Beckrow K (1999) Complementary therapy use among older cancer patients. Cancer Practice 7: 136–144.

CHAPTER 14

Dying

Time is too slow for those who wait, too swift for those who fear,
Too long for those who grieve, too short for those who rejoice,
But for those who love time is eternity.

Anon

This chapter explores ways in which complementary approaches can support traditional methods of nursing involved in the care of the dying and bereaved. Its aim is to help not only patients die a 'good' and dignified death but also to support relatives and carers during this time. Kubler-Ross (1968) referred to dying as 'the final stage of growth' or the culmination of the ageing process. Although the human experience of dying is uniquely individual, for all of us it is an inevitable part of life.

The aim therefore must be to help these individuals to adapt and participate in life as fully as possible until death occurs. As a result of enhanced technology there is, however, a danger that the dying process will become purely a medical event, physically and psychologically removed from both the family and associated community. Although there has been considerable discussion within the literature as to where is the most appropriate place to die, it is not within the remit of this chapter to enter this debate.

Many terms, such as journey, event or experience, are used to describe the commonalities of the dying process and the period of time between the realisation that death is imminent and the moment of death is often referred to as the 'dying trajectory'. This will, of course, be perceived individually by those concerned, but if this dying trajectory is long the patient may fear a painful death. Although 'natural death' (Hockley 1992) is rarely seen, many older people will still die without a terminal diagnosis and, although attitudes about death and dying appear now to be more open, there are still many associated taboos.

The practicalities of using aromatherapy, Bach flower remedies and massage

As the palliative care philosophy so mimics that espoused by complementary practitioners, it is appropriate to adopt it when discussing useful interventions. The palliative care approach aims to promote physical, psychosocial and spiritual well-being and enhance the quality of life of all involved (Letham 1999). It must be patient-centred and tailored to meet the patient's and relatives' constantly changing and complex needs wherever the patient is, whether at home, in residential care or nursing home or in hospital. But a recent joint survey by the *Nursing Times* and the Nuffield Trust (Addington-Hall 2001), which asked nurses 'How do you deal with death?', revealed some disturbing information. It found that a quarter of the respondents felt that the health service was failing to provide appropriate care for dying patients because there was often a lack of medical support or equipment to support this activity. Unfortunately, many of them also felt that pre- and post-registration education failed to provide them with the necessary skills to help such patients!

This may have dire consequences when considering quality-of-life issues because they are so very much influenced by the whole person approach, which needs to: take into account the person's past life experiences and current situation; provide care that involves both the dying person and those who matter to that person; respect patient autonomy and choice, e.g. over such things as the place of death and any treatment options; make available appropriate symptom control; and emphasise open and sensitive communication, which extends to patients, informal carers and professional colleagues alike.

But quality of life is extremely difficult to define. Lawton (1991) attempted to define it as:

> . . . the multi dimensional evaluation by both intra personal and social normative criteria of the person environment system.
>
> Laowton (1991)

But others have identified variables that people perceive are important to them and it is these that appear to affect or even predict an individual's quality of life. They include: financial status; having a network of friends; good quality family relationships; and decent living arrangements (Vetter et al. 1988). Choice, freedom and independence were also identified as influencing individuals' perceptions of their quality of life. In addition to these, they also felt that emotional well-being, which encompassed self-actualisation, self-esteem, self-worth and status, were vital. But all of these are potentially compromised in dying individuals.

Although each of these areas can be either objectively or subjectively measured, Felce and Perry (1995) stressed that it is essential to find out to what extent each domain is important to the individual being assessed because dilemmas may arise from these ideals in caring for dying patients, especially when one looks at issues relating to resources, treatments, variable environments of care and of course patients' choice in all of this!

Increasingly there seems to be a clear role emerging within complementary therapies to help the processes of dying and also bereavement. As a treatment they can provide an adjunct to more traditional ways and, although much of the literature appears to focus on patients dying of cancer, you can adapt treatment to reflect the individual needs of your patients. Where essential oils are used the most appropriate route must be chosen (see Chapter 4). Although there is great confusion in the literature about dilution strengths, where you are treating patients dying from cancer, low dilutions of between 1% (1 drop in 5 ml base oil) and 2.5% maximum are generally recommended. The lowest dilution should be used where patients are emotionally distraught or cachexic (see Chapter 13). Massage, if performed appropriately and sensitively, may be of great benefit to dying patients and their families (Gray 2000). Reflexology, strategically used, may help symptomatic management and also afford relaxation (see later for case study using reflexology as an adjunct to orthodox care). As many of the procedures and symptomatic treatments have been discussed elsewhere, I offer only new and specific information.

Bisset et al. (2001) feel that a sensible way of thinking about palliative care is to consider the notion of the 'dying spectrum'. At one end of the spectrum will be patients with:

> . . . relatively predictable and relentless diseases such as disseminated malignancy, [whilst] at the other are those with unpredictable, slowly progressing diseases such as multiple sclerosis or dementia. Between these extremes lie all those pathologies that may advance rapidly, kill unpredictably or respond in part to various treatments,

This implies a mammoth task, because all of these will need appropriate and effective management. The aims of treatment must therefore encompass initiatives that do the following.

Effect general relaxation

This has been considered in Chapters 10 and 12.

Palliation and symptom management

The prime focus here is to aid specific symptom control by offering practical supportive solutions in the treatment of the physical manifestations of disease, and also the side effects of orthodox treatments. As many of these have been considered in earlier chapters, I do not repeat the advice here, but instead consider a few pertinent interventions.

Nausea and vomiting

They are worthy of further discussion here because it has been estimated that 30% of terminally ill people experience vomiting and 60% experience nausea (Allan 1993). These often arise not only because of their illness, but also as a result of treatments and medication and their successful resolution remains a challenge (see Chapter 9 for treatment advice).

Constipation

This is also a considerable problem in terminal care, especially where opiate analgesia is used (see Chapter 9 for treatment).

Breathlessness and panic

Breathlessness is not always very well controlled by orthodox medication or oxygen therapy, and the resulting panic may require considerable skill to manage and measures either to control or to re-train breathing are often called for. Bailey (1997) stressed, however, that these would work only within a supporting forum where the sufferers could freely express their fears and worries. *Boswellia thurifera* (frankincense) is particularly useful here because it can slow and strengthen breathing, although it is also useful for those who are despondent (see Chapter 8 for other treatment).

Mouth care

Mennie (1997) noted that terminally ill individuals often experienced several oral problems. She stated that up to 89% of these patients harboured *Candida* species, but also suffered from other fungal infections, xerostomia and halitosis. As she was concerned that so many of the available mouth care products were not very effective in helping

these conditions, as part of her care of the dying coursework, she investigated the use of *Melaleuca alternifolia* (tea tree) as an alternative treatment.
Her clinical area has used it successfully ever since (see Chapter 9 for
other treatment).

Other symptoms include fungating wounds, anorexia, cough, insomnia, physical, emotional and spiritual (see below) pain and also pain associated with related conditions such as arthritis (see Chapter 13 and other
chapters).

Help deal with the individual's emotional responses which may surface at this time

These vary from individual to individual and will need expert skills to identify them accurately. Common ones are anxiety, grief (see below), sadness,
despondency, depression, frustration, fear and associated stresses. Some
special oils to use at this time are *Boswellia thurifera*, which helps despondency and lack of interest, and *Cananga odorata* (ylang ylang) and *Melissa
officinalis* (true melissa) because they are both calming and balancing, and
especially useful for those with anxiety, fear, depression, and unresolved
anger and frustration. Most of the Bach flower remedies would be suitable
to reduce emotional negativity and the choice would depend very much on
the emotion experienced (see Chapter 6 for the full list).

To foster hope?

Nurses have a key role in creating and fostering hope in dying individuals.
There is some evidence that the use of touch, discussed in earlier chapters, and the employment of listening skills and subsequent improvement
in the patient's self-worth, may encourage this. But it is also recognised
that nurses are mostly unaware of either the dying individual's need for
hope or the interventions that may optimise their hope levels.

Stephenson's (1991) definition:

> Hope is an anticipation, accompanied by desire and expectation of a positive, possible
> future . . .
>
> Stephenson (1991)

has often generalised improvement of the situation so that they see a
better future for themselves. But hope is a problematic concept because
it is difficult not only to define but also to measure or evaluate its
outcome. Sadly there is some debate about whether such skills can be
realistically used with dying patients, although Webb (1996) affirms that
any effective and caring relations need to build on a firm trusting

relationship that can be provided only by appropriately skilled and knowledgeable practitioners!

The concept of hope has been implicated in the process of adaptation and acceptance of chronic illness and death; Cutcliff (1996) notes that, even when nurses try to explore it, it is often too difficult to appreciate because hope is invariably poorly defined and described. Many definitions appear to neglect both the very importance of hope and also its individual nature. It is obvious, however, that hope is a very fragile entity and that its nurturing by most healthcare professionals tends to be subtle and implicit rather than overtly explicit, and in some cases is even ignored! Cutcliff (1996) does feel that there is a direct link between help and hope, and he suggests that the presence of a nurse carrying out everyday patient care may engender hope; Herth's (1990) work also suggests that a patient's potential is influenced by nurse activity. It may be helpful if we use therapies as a means of helping patients to regain some control of their dying journey, and help them to cope with not only the prognosis but also what lies ahead.

Herth (1990) emphasises that hope is not necessarily lost in the terminal stages of life and that the degree of hope that a patient may possess is not solely dependent on a poor prognosis. Although Herth (1990) does not address the consequences of the opposite concept of hopelessness, Herth feels that hope is essential to have all through life and to support the dying process. Although it is stressed that false hope should not be offered at this time, Ettinger (2001), a nurse chronicling her cancer journey in the *Nursing Times*, reckoned that a bit of 'false' hope was often better than no hope at all. Although much time is spent on physical assessments, often inadequate attention is paid to the psychological and spiritual needs of a patient.

Influence of spiritual belief, religion and the power of prayer and faith

There is some evidence that spiritual belief, which is not necessarily the same as religious conviction, although it sometimes encompasses this as well, may help seek meaning and perhaps hope out of the emotional turmoil at this time (Herth 1990, Ross 1994). Narayanasamy (1998) notes that spirituality tends to be less concrete and more subjective than religion because it has more to do with expression of our own inner personal feelings and experiences. Religion, on the other hand, is a more explicit and formal approach that appears to be influenced by external institutions and encompasses belief in a divine force, prayer and worship.

Although prayer does not belong exclusively to those who profess to be religious, it does often involve an attempt at 'speaking' to and asking for help from some divine power or God (Wright 2000). There is increasing evidence that prayer and faith are powerful aids to healing in some individuals and several studies have attempted to measure them.

Researchers (Koenig et al. 1997) at Duke University Medical Center in North Carolina (USA) sought to establish the potential interrelationships of religious activities, physical health and depressive symptoms and social support. Although the research yielded complex data, they found that frequency of church attendance correlated positively to physical health and negatively to depression. But they also found that bible and private prayer were negatively related to physical health. The researchers concluded that perhaps people prayed more when they needed help.

Other researchers (King and Bushwick 1994) in East Carolina (USA) had earlier sought to identify whether physicians asked patients about their religious beliefs. The survey noted that 68% of the patients said that they had never been asked about this and also 77% felt that the physician should do so. Interestingly 48% felt that their doctor should also pray with them.

Ross (1994), having identified that there were many studies that illustrated the relationship of belief and faith to health, sought to ascertain nurses' perceptions of spiritual care and how they identified and gave such care in practice. She found that many of those surveyed found it difficult to identify spiritual needs in patients who were unable to communicate fully. But a similar study by McSherry (1998) found that, although a large proportion of qualified nurses (71.4%) were able to identify patients with spiritual needs, only 39.9% of them felt that they could meet them. The barriers to this included not only time and resource issues, but also the belief, in some, that nurses should not be involved in such activities. Having said that, the majority of nurses did recognise that it was part of their role and were beginning to embrace more holistic concepts.

Spirituality is therefore apparently a nebulous concept and has been described as:

> . . . a quality that goes beyond religious affiliation, that strives for inspiration, reverence, awe, meaning and purpose, even in those who do not believe in any God. The spiritual dimension tries to be in harmony with the universe, strives for answers about the infinite, and comes into focus when the person faces emotional stress, physical illness or death.
>
> Murray and Zentner (1989)

According to Narayanasamy (1998) the expression of spirituality in older people is dependent on their upbringing and culture and at critical and stressful times, such as when dying, may act as a significant supporting mechanism that may help them come to terms with unresolved issues.

Oils that are deemed suitable to help create a spiritual environment and assist spiritual self-actualisation include *Rosa damascena* (rose), *Santalum album* (sandalwood), *Boswellia thurifera*, *Commiphora myrrha* (myrrh), *Citrus aurantium* (neroli), *Angelica archangelica* (angelica), *Jasminum officinale* (jasmine) and *Vetiveria zizanoides* (vetiver). *Helichrysum italicum* (or *Helichrysum immortelle*) is, however, seen by many as a sacred oil, which is supportive and comforting and allows safe reminiscence (Worwood 1999). But the oils will not provide this alone. Time is also required to allow dying people to reflect on their past life, reconcile some of their lost dreams and regrets, and forgive themselves for past occurrences. By affording them this opportunity for personal reflection, it may assist the transition from life to death.

Gamlin (1995) thought that, as hope was such a tenuous entity, even an unwitting comment could cause a person to lose hope. Unfortunately dying patients are not always told the truth in the belief that they will lose even more hope and die sooner. Sometimes the truth about their terminal diagnosis and prognosis may be withheld because either a professional carer or a relative feels that the patient will not be able to cope with such news. This paternalistic attitude may arise out of self-interest because relatives may have difficulty in coping with their imminent loss and health professionals may feel ill-equipped to deal with any issues arising from such honesty (Wright 1996). Although decisions relating to treatment and information giving have traditionally rested with medical staff, because of greater nurse expertise, autonomy and accountability, there has been a blurring of traditional nurse–doctor relationships. Nurses seem now more prepared to challenge some of these unitary decisions and initiate more collaborative practice, although caution is needed here. To challenge current practice, the nurse must be knowledgeable about such things and not compromise his or her duty of care.

Bereavement and the associated adjustment to this

Loss and grief

The process of grief is very individual and, in our rush to help people resolve it, Reoch (1998) urges that we do not impose our own beliefs and values on them. Therefore, where assistance is given, it should help people progress through the different stages and hopefully survive their grief journey. Although this progress through the various stages is not a linear one, it is important that these 'rites of passage' are encouraged at times of loss. Various authors have identified different bereavement processes, but it appears that there is no common definition for them or consensus of opinion as to how many there are (Stephen 1998). All are likely, however, to encompass feelings of shock, disbelief, denial, anger, remorse and adjustment. *Melissa officinalis*, which acts on the vital centres and helps balance delicate and fluctuating emotions and has been referred to as a remedy for the 'distressed spirit', is deemed to be essential to use at this time (Reoch 1998). Many of the Bach flower remedies and essential oils, previously discussed, will also be useful to treat the associated anxieties and symptoms.

The effects of being a carer (formal or informal)

Although it is advocated that trusts, etc. create and initiate strategies that will support carers, in reality it is often left to the individuals themselves to provide their own supportive mechanisms (Faulkner 1996). Although it is desirable to care for the carer in all areas of practice, within terminal care it is absolutely vital, because end-of-life care is so dependent on the care-givers coping with both the emotional and the physical traumas of the experience. One must remember, however, that carers will also be exposed to sudden, unexpected death and may be less prepared to cope with this. It would therefore be sensible if employing authorities provided complementary programmes not only for patients, but also for their workers as well (Faulkner 1996)!

There is considerable anecdotal evidence to support the notion that complementary therapies have a role to play in this support. One small study (Macdonald 1997) found that massage, as a respite intervention, was very useful in helping primary caregivers deal with the stresses of coping with their relatives and loved ones in the terminal situation. The study reported that the massage had reduced physical and emotional stress, pain and sleep disorders in most of the participants.

Reoch (1998) and Leigh (1998) both felt that lay carers would particularly benefit from some form of complementary therapy because the emotional and physical toil can be relentless and exhausting and is often with them 24 hours a day. Reoch (1998) suggested that caring should be a two-way affair and instead of carers just caring for the patient, the terminally ill patient should be encouraged to be more involved in the care of their carers. By doing this, they would still feel a valued member of their family. He also felt that this close relationship could be strengthened even further by both sides learning to massage each other's hands; then, instead of feeling helpless during the final stage together, they could create:

> ... an act of loving tenderness that [could] be expressed and shared when words fail. For people distressed by the suffering of a loved one, it offers a beautiful way to say with the warmth of human touch: 'I care for you deeply.'
>
> Reoch (1998)

To help coping

This is encompassed in the strategies discussed above.

To make the environment a more comfortable place

This can be done in a variety of ways. Deodorising essential oils such as *Cedrus atlantica* (cedarwood) could be used to mask offensive smells. The ambience could be enhanced by providing freshly cut, brightly coloured, perfumed flowers, or by the injection of sweet smells into the atmosphere by vaporising essential oils, burning incense or scented candles, via sachets of herbs or pot pourri. Personal fragrance and speciality bath blends or scented wash cloths could easily be made for the patient or carer by using oils that matched their individual needs. They could be used to elevate mood, calm the environment or foster a spiritual space (see above).

How would you create a soothing yet uplifting environment for your dying patient? Look again through the various chapters and Appendix I and identify what would be best provided in your particular area of practice.

Rebecca: a case study using reflexology as an adjunct to orthodox care

Initial visit

I was requested to visit the patient's ward by a student nurse because of the difficulty of easing her pain, despite careful positioning and large doses of diamorphine. Permission was sought and obtained from the patient's husband, her consultant and the ward manager. She looked very ill and shrivelled and was clearly a very frightened woman. She had wide staring eyes and was obviously cachexic but apyrexial. Although terminally ill, she was conscious and able to talk slowly but with some difficulty.

She was gently lifted into a semi-recumbent position, in bed, and she asked that Paul (the student nurse) stay with her while she was treated. He helped her maintain this position. Some time was spent on introductions and her medical history was obtained from the student nurse and her case notes.

Patient background and current problems

Rebecca was a 69-year-old, terminally ill patient, confined to bed on an acute surgical ward. She had suffered from lung cancer for 5 years, had completed her radiotherapy over a year ago, but recent investigation showed further carcinoma infiltration in both lungs with bony metastases. Although on large doses of diamorphine, administered continually via a syringe driver, she was still experiencing intractable pain. She was also on regular night sedation and aperients and antiemetics as required. She appeared very emaciated and was receiving a liquidised diet with some oral supplementation. Her urinary output was sparse, and oral and rectal aperients mostly controlled her bowels.

Visual examination

Her feet were white and cold with patches of redness on both outer aspects of her ankles and around her heels. The skin was yellow and mottled on the dorsum in the lung area. She was noticeably tender in the solar plexus. Initially I spent quite a while gently effleuraging and moving her feet. (She had not stood for quite a few days.) I made a cursory examination of the reflex zones of both feet. It seemed appropriate to massage only the adrenals and solar plexus to help her pain and stress. I also attempted to stimulate the reddened areas, which included the hip area. In addition, I paid some attention to the lymphatic drainage points. I spent approximately 30 minutes touching her feet.

After treatment

Paul asked to bathe and apply scented talc to her feet. I wrote the treatment in her nursing notes. In addition, I asked that her feet be positioned carefully and that any pressure on them be relieved. I also asked that she be encouraged to drink more. Paul agreed to report any changes in the patient.

Second visit

I returned to this patient 4 days later, and noticed that her care plan stated that, although her pain did not appear totally resolved, she was restful. On examination her feet were cool, she had no redness around the ankles or heels, but the dorsum was still very yellow. She was tender in the solar plexus, so I gently massaged these areas, and also made contact with her adrenals. This time I felt more confident to work on the lung area, including the bronchus, and also tried to stimulate the spine. I hoped that this would help her bony pain. Her hip and pelvic area was stimulated and I briefly contacted the ovarian areas again on the outer aspects of her ankles. Again all points were covered. She was more receptive on this occasion and asked me to visit again.

Third visit

This time I saw the patient alone as she was sitting out in the chair. I observed that there was no redness over any bony prominences and that her feet now had a pink tinge except in the lung area. I treated the same areas as on the second visit but also investigated further the urinary tract and intestinal regions.

Fourth visit

Rebecca had asked a nurse to contact me to visit her because she felt the reflex stimulation provided some pain relief. This time I used extremely gentle techniques, as I was afraid to over-stimulate her. She responded well and talked about her husband and two children. Her feet were again very white but she was very relaxed.

Fifth visit

The following day I was informed that Rebecca had lost consciousness. I sat with her husband who asked me to 'rub' her feet. This was difficult because she was on her side and it was not appropriate to move her. A nurse helped hold her feet and I gently effleuraged and made contact (hopefully) with the head areas and adrenals to help her pain relief.

Postscript

Sadly, over the following weekend Rebecca died. She never regained consciousness, but died peacefully. I was reluctant to use her as a case study, but her husband requested that I did.

Death is a difficult subject to confront because it is still surrounded by sacred and ill-informed taboos. Although complementary therapies cannot provide answers for these, they do give dying patients and their careers other options to explore. By using them within existing health structures, they also have the potential to add another dimension to the support of patients in their quest to live meaningfully until they die! But remember:

> Death is nothing at all – I have only slipped away into the next room – I am I and you are you, whatever we were to each other, that we are still. Call me by my old familiar name speak to me in the easy way which you always used. Put no differences in your tone; wear no false air of solemnity or sorrow. Laugh as we always laughed at the little jokes we enjoyed together. Play, smile, think of me, pray for me. Let my name be forever the household word that it always was. Let it be spoken without effect, without the ghost of a shadow on it. Life means all that it ever meant. It is the same as it ever was: there is absolutely unbroken continuity. What is this death but a negligible accident? Why should I be out of mind because I am out of sight? I am waiting for you, for an interval, somewhere very near, just around the corner , . . . All is well.
>
> Henry Scott Holland (1847–1918)

Learning activity

- To be able to give effective care you need to be physically and emotionally well, so how will you support, comfort and protect yourself at this time?
- Identify your individual needs and then, using the philosophies discussed in this book, devise a personal programme that will assist your own 'therapeutic healing' and help you to remain calm, focused and professionally fulfilled.
- Are there others in your working or home environment that could also benefit from such a programme?

References

Addington-Hall J (2001) The end results. Nursing Times 97(21): 24–25.

Allan S (1993) Nausea and vomiting. In: Doyle D, Hanks G, McDonald N, eds, Oxford Textbook of Palliative Medicine. Oxford: Oxford University Press .

Bailey C (1997) Professional development. Breathlessness. Nursing Times 1(6): 5–8.

Bisset M, Robinson R, George R (2001) Expanding the remit of palliative care. Nursing Times 97(21): 38–40.

Cutcliff J (1996) Critically ill patients' perspectives of hope. British Journal of Nursing 5(11): 674, 687–690.

Ettinger F (2001) Faith in healers. Nursing Standard 15(32): 26.

Faulkner A (1996) Care of oncology patients: caring for the carers. Complementary Therapies in Nursing and Midwifery 2: 59–61.

Felce D, Perry J (1995) Quality of life: its definition and measurement. Research in Developmental Disabilities 16: 51–74.

Gamlin R (1995) Using hope to cope with loss and grief. Nursing Standard 9(48): 33–35.

Gray R (2000) The use of massage therapy in palliative care. Complementary Therapies in Nursing and Midwifery 6: 77–82.

Herth K (1990) Fostering hope in terminally ill people. Journal of Advanced Nursing 15: 1250–1259.

Hockley J (1992) Death and dying. In: Redfern S, ed., Nursing Elderly People. Edinburgh: Churchill Livingstone.

King D, Bushwick B (1994) beliefs and attitudes about faith healing and prayer. Journal of the Family Practitioner 39: 349–352.

Koenig H, Hays J, George L et al. (1997) Modeling the cross-sectional relationships between religion, physical health, social support and depressive symptoms. American Journal of Geriatric Psychiatry 5: 131–144.

Kubler-Ross E (1968) On Death and Dying. London: Tavistock.

Lawton M (1991) A multi-dimensional view of quality of life in frail elders. In: Binen J, Lubben J, Rose J, Deutchman D, eds, The Concept and Measurement of Quality of Life in the Frail Elderly. New York: Academic Press: 3–27.

Leigh H (1998) Aromatherapy in terminal care. The Aromatherapist 5(2):18–26.

Letham W (1999) Nursing home nurses deliver palliative care. Nursing Times 95(44): 54–55.

Macdonald G (1997) Massage as an alternative respite intervention for primary caregivers of the terminally ill. Alternative Therapies in Clinical Practice 4(3): 86–89.

McSherry W (1998) Nurses' perceptions of spirituality and spiritual care. Nursing Standard 13(4): 36–40.

Mennie A (1997) An essential and ancient oil. Nursing Times 93(47): 41–42.

Murray R, Zentner J (1989) Nursing Concepts for Health Promotion. New York: Prentice Hall.

Narayanasamy A (1998) Religious and spiritual needs of older people. In: Pickering S, Thompson J, eds, Promoting Positive practice in Nursing Older People: Perspectives on Quality of Life. London: Baillière Tindall.

Reoch R (1998) Dying well: the holistic approach. The Aromatherapist 5(2): 27–33.

Ross L (1994) Spiritual care: the nurse's role. Nursing Standard 8(29): 33–37 .

Stephen R (1998) Aromatherapy and bereavement (for the aromatherapist). The Aromatherapist 5(2): 8–16.

Stephenson C (1991) The concept of hope revisited for nursing. Journal of Advanced Nursng (16) 1456–1461.

Vetter N, Jones DA, Victor CR (1998) The quality of life of the over 70's in the community. Health Visitor 61: 10–13.

Webb C (1996) Caring, curing, coping: towards an integrated model. Journal of Advanced Nursing 23: 960–968.

Worwood V (1988) The Fragrant Heavens. London: Transworld Publishers Ltd.

Wright B (1996) Sudden Death: A research base for practice, 2nd edn. New York: Churchill Livingstone.

Wright S (2000) Praying for good health. Nursing Standard 15(2): 27.

Further reading

Abel J (2000) Complementary therapy programme at St Luke's Hospice, Plymouth. Complementary Therapies in Nursing and Midwifery 6: 116–119.

Anderson J, Anderson L, Felsenthal G (1993) Pastoral needs and support within an inpatient rehabilitation unit. Archives of Physical Medicine and Rehabilitation 74: 574–578.

Cadwallader M (1998) Complementary healing modalities and their use in palliative care. The Aromatherapist 5(2): 44–47.

Evans B (1995) An audit into the effects of aromatherapy massage and the cancer patient in palliative and terminal care. Complementary Therapies in Medicine 3: 239–241.

Hinton J (1967) Dying. London: Penguin.

Howard J (1990) The Bach Flower Remedies Step by Step. Saffron Walden: CW Daniel Co. Ltd.

Kinghorn S (1995) Easing patient discomfort. Nursing Times 91(34): 57–59 .

Lynch N (1997) Cold comfort. Nursing Times 93(37): 42–43.

Millar B (1998) Palliative care for people with non-malignant disease. Nursing Times 94(48): 52–53.

Miller R (1996) The use of aromatherapy in hospitals for patients with cancer. The Aromatherapist 3(2): 14–29.

Narayanasamy A (1998) Religious and spiritual needs of older people. Cited in Pickering and Stephensen (1991).

Penson J (1998) Complementary therapies: making a difference in palliative care. Complementary Therapies in Nursing and Midwifery 4: 77 81.

Pickering S, Thompson J (1991) The concept of hope revisited for nursing. Journal of Advanced Nursing 16: 1456–1461.

Walker S (1997) Intercessory prayer: a pilot investigation funded by the Office of Alternative Medicine. Alternative Therapies in Medicine 3(2): 104–105.

Wilson V (1999) Meeting the needs of dying patients and their carers. Journal of Community Nursing 13(9): 26–34.

CHAPTER 15

The way forward

There is danger that the phenomenon may, like the butterfly that is pinned down for closer inspection, be destroyed in the attempts to understand it.

Janet Quinn (1995)

This chapter aims to draw together the themes of this book and establish how far we have come on this complementary journey. It then offers ideas about what still needs to be pursued so that patients and nurses may be able to exercise some choice in the use of complementary approaches. Before we can move forward, however, it is necessary to understand some of the constraining arguments and influences impeding nurses in this.

Orthodox medicine versus complementary therapies

There is a huge debate currently within both the nursing and the medical literature about the advantages of one system over the other. All appear to have a vested interest in promoting their particular style of therapy rather than helping their patients, as the linchpin in all of this, to make informed choices about what is on offer. Whether this is helpful in making complementary therapies more acceptable and available remains to be seen.

Davis (1997) notes how traditional medical practice is still seen as the only valid approach to curing disease or injury and suggests that having to consider other treatment rationales will necessarily involve a paradigmatic shift away from a linear hierarchical approach to a more holistic non-linear integrated approach. She says that orthodox medicine has just become the preferred way of knowing and that complementary therapies could be legitimised if their safety and efficacy could be established.

Vickers (1999) feels, however, that complementary therapists are not only often openly antagonistic towards conventional medicine, but also disparaging about its achievements. He feels that the most common misinformation that complementary therapists give is the example that their work is holistic and medicine is not. He goes on to challenge the validity of such practitioners questioning the worth of medicine when they may have no knowledge about orthodox practice. And yet it is just this that orthodox practitioners do about alternative practice, often with no or very little knowledge! He ends his somewhat hostile article by saying that as the patients' well-being is the prime consideration of all practitioners, they should respect each other's viewpoint and be willing to collaborate for the benefit of the patient!

Kendrick (1999), a very astute political writer, stated that complementary therapies have over the last 20 years re-emerged as an adjunct to traditional Western medicine and that this has afforded nurses many opportunities to embrace these newer skills and so offer patients a choice of different therapies. He added that, although nurses have been keen to do this, orthodox medicine has been concerned over safety issues and their lack of supposed scientific rigour. He clearly feels that medicine is threatened by the competition that the introduction of complementary therapies has posed. He is also extremely critical of how doctors have been portrayed as all knowing and also believes that this clinical power has not only inhibited the development of nursing, but also constrained individuals from embarking on unorthodox practices, because they have made such innovative practice so politically sensitive.

Like Davis (1997), Kendrick also refers to the paradigm shift and, although recognising that the challenges that lie ahead to achieve this are immense, he feels that the benefits of offering more choice to patients outweighs the difficulties. He asserts that, instead of just acquiescing to this unequal medical power base, we should attempt to develop a non-utopian working relationship between all of the various healthcare professionals, so that our prime aim is the enrichment of healthcare provision.

In an anonymous article (Anon 2000), it has been noted that the climate within medicine in response to patients' use of complementary and alternative practice may be changing. The issue of how orthodox medical practitioners respond to or even integrate complementary medicine into their work is ever more pressing. And those clinical questions raise the further matter of evaluating complementary practice. Before doctors rush to condemn the evidence base underpinning these therapies, they should pause and consider the record of orthodox medicine.

This article gives examples of how orthodox drugs have been withdrawn from the market and notes also how the procedures employed for evaluating the safety and efficacy of drugs, regarded as products of scientific Western medicine, are, at best, imperfect.

The author notes that, although the Report of the House of Lords' Select Committee on Science and Technology (2000) into complementary and alternative medicine found that 'quality control across complementary methods is poor' in relation to practitioner training, safety and efficacy, it did recognise that some complementary medicines were worthy of serious consideration. This article then stated that this was possibly more to do with the general public's continued endorsement of them, rather than any medical influence. It advocated that the time was now ripe for unorthodox therapies to be subjected to more rigorous analysis, but at the same time asserted that the standards for evaluating orthodox medicine were also open to question.

It has been suggested that double standards exist in judging traditional versus complementary approaches because a high percentage of medical practice is not scientifically proven or even shown to do more good than harm. Indeed Dr Ian Chalmers (1998), the Director of the UK Cochrane Centre, and a vigorous proponent of systematic reviews, noted that not all orthodox medical practices were well evaluated. He recounted how the physician Van Helmont had questioned the rationale behind the orthodox practice of bloodletting more than 350 years ago. He asserted also that, although medicine has helped people to live longer over the last 50 years, sometimes its confidence in itself is misplaced. He also felt that it was important for critics of complementary medicine to be aware that allopathic medicine has a 'far greater potential for causing widespread harm' than individual complementary interventions. This is because they are normally more potent and also used more widely.

Critics of complementary approaches are often far more assiduous in their attempts to outlaw unevaluated complementary practices than unevaluated orthodox practices. As so many people turn to them, in the belief that they are effective, he believes, however, that it is essential to assess them thoroughly by the use of controlled trials. Only then will people be able to make informed choices about any given therapy. He acknowledges and pays tribute to therapists who are embarking on this journey and feels that an integrated medical system will be a reality only if all practitioners are truly humble and recognise that:

. . . good intentions, plausible theories and strong beliefs about the benefits of treatments, orthodox or complementary, provide no guarantee that they will do more good
than harm.

Chalmers (1998)

Alongside this growth in the popularity of complementary approaches
to care, there is, undoubtedly, a growing need to develop a rigorous, systematic and sustained evidence base. Much of the criticism levelled at complementary practitioners, by orthodox medicine, is associated with increasing
anxiety about treatment efficacy and safety. These criticisms, however, also
coincide with the increasingly empirical world of medicine, and the value
placed on randomised controlled trials (RCTs). Although there is a desire in
some areas to promote the use of RCTs in complementary therapies, and
such an approach is admirable, it is important to step back and consider
whether these are the right measures to assess the needs of this area of practice adequately. Often this debate only reflects two diametrically opposed
arguments. It is asserted, on the one hand, that because conventional medicine is scientifically based it can deliver safe and effective treatments and,
on the other, that complementary therapies have little or no research base
to support safe practice. Yet orthodox medicine itself has often been based
on the prevailing culture, anecdotal beliefs, and custom and practice, and is
only now beginning to discover empiricism.

It is apparent then, that although complementary practice must
acknowledge problems in relation to systematic evidence and regulation,
which are both crucial to its integration into mainstream clinical practice,
it is still judged harshly by those who perhaps fear its growing popularity.
The call for the same systematic research approaches has come from both
sides of the debate, but clearly reliable tools are needed for both
approaches, and the most appropriate methodology regarding outcomes
and effectiveness needs to be considered in relation to the therapeutic
modality offered.

Le May (1999), although not writing purely about complementary
therapies, noted that there is growing unease about the 'narrow, research-
dominated interpretation of evidence' because she believes that practice
should be informed by as many sources as possible.

Although not advocating a return to the 'cookbook' approach to nursing care, she suggests that we adopt flexible approaches which enable us
to unearth appropriate evidence on which to base best practice. She
believed that the following sources could be an effective way of 'building
up' a diverse evidence base:

- Orthodox type research: this could include original research papers and literature reviews.
- Experiential (evidence): this would involve reflecting on practice and using non-research literature, narratives and case studies.
- Non-research-based theory: this could involve looking at published and unpublished literature, and using information learnt from another, e.g. from classroom information provided by a teacher.
- Data from patients/clients/carers: this may include both research and non-research-based evidence, experiential writings and qualitative audit material.
- Role model 'expert experience': here information may come from evaluations, expert opinion, discussion and observation.
- Policy directives: these could be both published and unpublished, local and national clinical guidelines, and standards of care.

When appraising non-researched work, in order to maintain clinical credibility and competence, it is essential that the quality of the work is considered and for what reason it was written, e.g. if a wheelchair manufacturer wrote a book on disability and old age, the evidence might be extremely useful, but the author may have a 'vested interest' to write this because it may increase the sales of his product!

A further significant difficulty for research in the field of complementary therapies is the lack of financial support because within the UK it is often difficult to obtain. Ernst (1999) reported that, in 1996, only 0.08% of funding for research in the NHS went to complementary therapies. Furthermore, although the Medical Research Council (MRC) has an annual research budget of approximately £319 million and despite seven applications, it chose to fund only one related research study between 1994 and 1999. Such funding could also compromise original research because it mostly comes from the charitable donations or tax contributions made by the general public. As a result of this it is often spent according to the donors' wishes and not necessarily according to need.

He felt that other nations might inform our future strategies, because many of them have supported centres of excellence by ring fencing money for research. The European Commission Cost Action B4 (1998) report on unconventional medicine supports the above need for research and advises that it might best be achieved by a combined European strategy rather than single nation initiatives.

The greatest concern of complementary therapists with regard to the scientific approach is that it is likely to compromise their therapeutic integrity and would just produce another medicalised therapy. However, there is a responsibility placed on us as professionals to promote safe and effective best practice. We need also to ensure that patients have appropriate information so that they may make informed decisions about the safety and efficacy of any therapy they wish to access. Having said this, Wood (1998), an orthodox biochemist, questions why practitioners of these therapies need to incorporate research activity, beyond simple practice audit into their practice, when patients keep flocking to see them.

Although biomedicine's 'claim to validity' is its scientific diagnostic base, it seems that even this is only socially constructed, because even diagnosis is influenced by cultural norms and expectations (Hopwood 1997). As a result of this he says that medical intervention should be viewed only as just one of the many differing healing systems that patients may choose to adopt. Although we may be concerned about the safety and validity of some of the other therapies on offer, he asks whether we have the right to preclude patients from using them. He gives the following example from Foster and Anderson's (1978) anthropological writings:

> For jaundice, mix powdered frozen potatoes with three lice and the urine of a black cow, and drink the potion on Tuesdays and Fridays.
>
> Foster and Anderson (1978)

But will such illustrations add credibility to our current debate because it seems to portray an unrealistic and scary 'New Age' quackery image? Some current media headlines, even in the quality press, do this. *The Times* (1999) in its features spread (page 17) had two particularly emotive headlines that stood out:

> 'Sceptic seeks New Age Therapy' and 'Spin your throat chakra in a clockwise direction'. Eh?
>
> *The Times* (March 1999)

This image has also been compounded by the trivial and damaging tone and inadequate knowledge expressed in two articles published in the *Nursing Standard* (Rayner 1999a) and *Nursing Times* (Rayner 1999b) by this celebrated 'Agony Aunt' and one-time nurse. They provoked a huge response from nurses and caused an absolute furore in the succeeding weeks' letters page of both journals.

The nurses' role in the integration of complementary therapies into orthodox care

It has been indicated that, as nurses are already *in situ* as carers for patients, they would be the ones best suited to carry out complementary therapies. This may be very unrealistic, currently, because of all the other claims made on their time. However, nurses are in a unique position to 'spur on' other health professionals towards a more patient-centred approach to care, as effective change agents (Wright 1989).

Johnson (2000) questioned, however, whether nurses should actually practise complementary therapies. Her literature review suggested that there was no evidence to show that nurses practising complementary therapies got better results with patients than complementary practitioners, especially when these practitioners were more skilled than they were. When nurses did practise them, the choice of therapy practised seemed to be correlated to both the cost and the length of study time involved, and the acceptability of the therapy to other professionals and themselves. She concluded that, although there may be a place for complementary therapies within nursing, they should be practised according to the needs of patients and not those of the nurses.

It seems that, at times, it may be preferable to use specialist practitioners, rather than nurses, to provide such care. The creation of a partnership approach between all concerned would, however, seem eminently sensible to adopt because nurses do not and should not have exclusive rights over any patient! This is very pertinent to consider because, when nurses are using complementary therapies with their patients, they are often only 'borrowing' some of the expert skills or tasks from these practitioners and may also rely somewhat heavily on them to help achieve this (Avis 1999, Brett 1999).

Chadwick (1999), as part of her Master of Science degree, sought to elicit the reasoning behind nurses' desires to practise complementary therapies. Within her survey, which accessed information from all over the country, she added four specific subquestions. These asked if the use of therapies was:

... for the enhancement of care delivered, to promote autonomous practice, 'breaking' away from the medical dominance or to support role expansion?

Chadwick (1999)

She was amazed by the results because she had expected that enhancing patient care and moving away from medical dominance would have scored most highly, but the question about role expansion achieved this. The fact that nurses were choosing to take on things more for themselves, as opposed to enhancing patients' care, very much supports what Johnson (2000) had concluded. After reflecting on her small-scale study, she (Chadwick 1999) could identify with this because of the current pressures on nurses to justify their role.

Wright (1995) asserts that the future route for nurses practising such therapies may be beset with difficulties and advocates that we should be competent to practise these skills safely. Stuttard and Walker (2000) support this thinking and feel that any education should start within pre-registration programmes, so that the students are able to support enhanced nursing models and:

> ... uphold the challenge of integrating orthodox and complementary approaches to care in the future.
>
> Stuttard and Walker (2000)

Wright (1995) further demands that we select reputable training courses, embrace self-development opportunities so that we may:

> ..., marry the scientific with the intuitive to produce the research that supports our case, to build the knowledge and skills that are needed to live in this reality while pursuing the vision of the next. Nurses have often felt themselves buffeted by the will and actions of others. [He asks] will it be different this time?
>
> Wright (1995)

The report below is likely to influence all of this.

The House of Lords Report

The sixth report from the House of Lords Select Committee on Science and Technology on Complementary and Alternative Medicine (CAM) (2000) may have a huge influence on the future practice of many of the therapies that have been discussed in this book. This report, which received more than 180 written submissions and took evidence from 46 different bodies, was produced after a 15-month enquiry. The key points are presented below.

The Committee reported that, because the use of complementary and alternative medicine was now so widespread and increasing within the industrialised West, there were likely to be many issues for future health policy-makers to address. These would include matters concerning the evidence base and regulation of the therapies themselves and the status and education of those who would provide them. Although they recognised that some of the therapies had either satisfactorily accomplished this or were about to, they commented that many had not.

CAMs include a vast assortment of therapies and the committee proposed that they be divided into the following three therapies:

- Group 1: they identified these as being complete systems of assessment and treatment and within this they included the most organised professions, 'The Big Five' therapies of chiropractic, homoeopathy, osteopathy, acupuncture and herbal medicine, because they concluded that they had some research-based evidence to support their effectiveness. Therapies within this group are thought to be likely to be responsive to research and appear to have already done so to a substantial degree. The opportunities for provision of these, in the NHS, is ever increasing.

- Group 2 contains those therapies that most clearly complement conventional medical treatment with the use of various supportive techniques and include the Alexander technique, aromatherapy, bodywork therapies such as massage and shiatsu, reflexology and hypnotherapy. The NHS is already providing these therapies for specialist care, such as terminal, palliative care, and have already encouraged and embarked on research activity into the efficacy of many of their treatments. Many of the individual organisations concerned with these therapies are currently addressing issues in relation to training and regulation as well as research and some will amalgamate to help this process.

- Group 3 comprised those therapies that, although they were long-established and traditional systems of health care, were not deemed to have a convincing evidence base. These included: Ayurvedic medicine, an ancient Indian discipline which uses natural herbs in treatments; Chinese herbal medicine and traditional Chinese medicine (TCM), which both use unorthodox treatments and diagnostic techniques; crystal therapy which as its name suggests uses crystals to 'fine tune' the body's energy patterns; iridology which treats problems by studying the iris of both eyes; and dowsing which is used as a way of answering questions intuitively during other complementary treatments. Although the report recognised their longstanding application in many other cultures, it felt that they could not be supported unless and until convincing research evidence showing efficacy, based on the results of well-designed trials, could be produced. For therapies in group 3, the prospect of attracting research funding or being provided within NHS settings remains improbable. There has been tremendous debate and unrest within the therapies concerned about this.

The main conclusions of the report

To protect the public from the potential risks of poor complementary practice the report advocated that there needed to be:

1. Improved and robust regulatory systems set up for all therapies.
2. Adequate education and training, via standardised, validated and accredited programmes – where nurses were intending to use them in their practice, the UKCC (or new statutory body) should develop specific competencies and guidelines for them. Opportunities for continuing education and updating of practice should be forthcoming.
3. Cohesive strategies for research and opportunities for training in this. The report also advocated that a central mechanism to advise on and coordinate CAM research would be advisable. There should also be ring-fenced money from central government for these activities.
4. A central unbiased source of clear and effective information about the efficacy and availability of treatments for potential users. Such users should be encouraged not to miss out on conventional medicine. It also said that it would be unfair to deter patients from seeking other treatments, although only those with an established evidence base could attract financial support.
5. More integration and open-mindedness between CAM and orthodox medicine so that patients have the opportunity to be helped by both, through cross-referral.

It will be interesting to watch how all of this unfolds!

Botting and Cook (2000), when reviewing studies involving doctors and in particular general practitioners' views about the use of and attitudes towards CAM, said it was vital to be aware of these because of the clinical control that they are able to exert over patients and nurses alike. This twofold power may prevent patients being referred to other practitioners and, because of their clinical authority over patients, may decide whether or not a nurse may use any of the therapies with their patients. Unfortunately many of these decisions are often made with wilfully inadequate knowledge about the therapies that are being practised!

Perhaps the time is now ripe for complementary and orthodox medicine to come closer together and provide a united and integrated healthcare service. Although it appears to be an attractive proposition, how feasible would it be? Trevelyan (1998) noted that the NHS Confederation study in 1996 found that, although many complementary therapies are now found in most NHS settings and that they offered a range of 'perceived benefits' to patients, their integration into practice settings was often hindered. The study found that this was often the result of a lack of funds or interest to support these initiatives, especially when information about the effectiveness and supporting rationale behind these therapies or where to find competent practitioners was lacking. As senior managers were also said to be unenthusiastic, anyone seeking to introduce such measures had to fight harder for a slice of the limited resources.

As the moves towards using complementary therapies alongside allopathic medicine is so patently public led, it seems sensible to consider that a truly integrated therapeutic service can be practised honourably by all parties only if the issues raised in the Foundation for Integrated Medicine (FIM 1997) and House of Lords (2000) reports are funded and supported in a collaborative manner by all health professionals and Government alike. Undoubtedly, nurses must be prepared to undertake more research into complementary therapies to enhance their credibility in practice and satisfy the medical profession and management of the benefits to patients, because it seems obvious that purchasers will not allocate any of their budgets to unproven therapies.

The way forward must be to provide a service where all patients can benefit from the best of both worlds, where they can exercise choice and be able to use orthodox treatments alongside the unconventional therapies if desired. The onus is on all nurses to discover all they can about complementary therapies so that they may influence their provision knowledgeably, because to withhold their potential benefits from patients is unethical and could even be illegal (Dimond 1997). How near are we to this ideal?

I must reassure you that this book was not written with a view to dissuading you from trying to integrate chosen therapies into your areas of practice. But I can promise you that, unless you are fully committed to the idea, the lengthy consultation and implementation period required may deter you from implementing even minor changes!

Study activity

Having contemplated the above evidence, where will you go from here?

References

Anon (2000) Complementary medicine: time for critical engagement. The Lancet **356**: 2023.

Avis A (1999) When is an aromatherapist not an aromatherapist? Complementary Therapies in Nursing and Midwifery **7**: 116–118.

Brett H (1999) Aromatherapy in the care of older people. Nursing Times **95**(33): 56–57.

Botting D, Cook R (2000) Complementary medicine: knowledge, use and attitudes of doctors. Complementary Therapies in Nursing and Midwifery **6**: 41–47.

Chadwick L (1999) What are the reasons for nurses using complementary therapy in practice. Complementary Therapies in Nursing and Midwifery 5: 144–148.

Chalmers I (1998) Evidence of the effects of health care: a plea for a single standard across 'orthodox' and 'complementary' medicine. Complementary Therapies in Medicine 6: 211–212.

Davis C, ed. (1997) Complementary Therapies in Rehabilitation: Holistic approaches for prevention and wellness. Thorofare, NJ: Slack Inc.

Dimond B (1997) Questions and answers on the legal aspects of complementary therapy. Complementary Therapies in Nursing and Midwifery 3: 156–159.

Ernst E (1999) Funding research into complementary medicine: the situation in Britain. Complementary Therapies in Medicine 7: 250–253.

European Commission Cost Action B4 (1998) Unconventional Medicine: Final report of the management committee 1993–1998. EUR 18420 EN.

Foundation for Integrated Medicine (1997) Integrated Health Care: A way forward for the next five years. London: FIM.

Foster G, Anderson B (1978) Medical anthropology. Cited in Hopwood (1997).

Hopwood A (1997) The social construction of illness and its implications for complementary and alternative medicine. Complementary Therapies in Medicine 5: 152–155.

House of Lords Select Committee on Science and Technology (2000) The 6th Report on Complementary and Alternative Medicine (HL Paper 123). London: The Stationery Office (www.publications.parliament.uk).

Johnson G (2000) Should nurses practise complementary therapies? Complementary Therapies in Nursing and Midwifery 6: 120–123.

Kendrick K (1999) Challenging power, autonomy and politics in complementary therapies: a contentious view. Complementary Therapies in Nursing and Midwifery 5: 77–81.

Le May (1999) Evidence-based Practice. Nursing Times Clinical Monographs 1. London: NT Books, Emap Healthcare Ltd.

Rayner C (1999a) Perspectives: opinion. Stuff and nonsense. Nursing Standard 13(3): 22–23.

Rayner C (1999b) Hot potatoes. Opiate of the people. Nursing Times 95(32: 30–31.

Stuttard P, Walker E (2000) Integrating complementary therapy into the nursing curriculum. Complementary Therapies in Nursing and Midwifery 6: 87–90.

The Times (1999) Features. The Times March 12.

Trevelyan J (1998) Complementary therapies on the NHS: current practice, future development (Part 1). Complementary Therapies in Nursing and Midwifery 4: 82–84.

Vickers A (1999) Editorial. Complementary medicine or antagonistic medicine? Complementary Therapies in Medicine 7: 125.

Wood C (1998) Do therapists need to do research? Complementary Therapies in Medicine 6: 208–210.

Wright S, ed. (1989) Changing Nursing Practice. London: Edward Arnold.

Wright S (1995) Bringing the heart back into nursing. Complementary Therapies in Nursing and Midwifery 1: 15–20.

Further reading

Baker S (2001) AOC update. Aromatherapy World: Seeding March 4.

Le May (1999) Evidence-based Practice. Nursing Times Clinical Monographs 1. London: NT Books, Emap Healthcare Ltd.

APPENDIX I
Essential oils

The essential oils are presented under their common names in order that they may easily be recognised. In each case their Latin botanical names are given alongside so that their plant genus and species may be readily identified. Please note that all essential oils have the potential for misuse and unsafe handling. They should therefore be kept out of the reach of children or other vulnerable populations, stored in cool dark places, never taken internally or applied to the skin neatly and the recommended dose should not be exceeded (see Appendix II for list of hazardous oils).

Benzoin (*Styrax benzoin*)

Principal properties: anti-infectious, anxiolytic, diuretic, emotional, expectorant, immunostimulant, skin care, tonic, warming
Treatment route: bath, inhalation and massage
Specific contraindications: none known
Countries of origin: Sumatra
Note: base
Blends well with rose

Bergamot (*Citrus bergamia*)

Principal properties: aphrodisiac, antidepressant, anti-infectious, anti-septic, calming, sedative, skin care
Treatment route: bath, compress, inhalation and massage
Specific contraindications: none known, should not be used neat on the skin or applied before sunbathing as this oil may cause photosensitivity of the skin

Countries of origin: Morocco, West Africa, Italy, Guinea
Note: top
Blends well with most oils

Black pepper (*Piper nigrum*)

Principal properties: analgesic, antibacterial, antifungal, antimicrobial, antiseptic, carminative, digestive, diuretic, expectorant, laxative, rubefacient, stimulant, tonic, warming
Specific contraindications: none known, use moderately as it may cause skin irritation and increase phototoxicity
Countries of origin: India, Indonesia, China, Malaysia, Madagascar
Note: Middle
Blends well with: frankincense, sandalwood, lavender, rosemary and marjoram

Cajuput (*Melaleuca leucadendron*)

Principal properties: analgesic, antibacterial, antiseptic, antispasmodic, decongestant, digestive, expectorant, sudorific
Treatment route: bath, compress, inhalation and massage
Specific contraindications: none known, may irritate sensitive skin
Countries of origin: Indonesia, Malaysia
Note: top
Blends well with: lavender

Clary sage (*Salvia sclarea*)

Clary sage is deemed safer than sage by many aromatherapists.
Principal properties: antifungal, anti-spasmodic, detoxicant, euphoric, hormonal, neurotonic, regenerative, sedative, tonic
Treatment route: bath, compress, inhalation and massage
Specific contraindications: alcohol and clary sage used together may precipitate a headache or nightmare, not normally used with cancer sufferers
Countries of origin: Spain, France
Note: top/middle
Blends well with bergamot, geranium, juniper, lavender, rose and sandalwood

Fennel (*Foeniculum vulgare*)

Principal properties: analgesic, antibacterial, anti-inflammatory, carminative, circulatory stimulant, decongestant, detoxifying, digestive, eliminative, emmenagogue, hormonal, laxative, oestrogenic, skin care
Treatment route: bath, compress, inhalation and massage
Specific contraindications: safe in normal doses but high doses may cause disturbance of the nervous system, considered unsafe to use in cases of epilepsy, avoided in children and pregnancy
Countries of origin: Japan, India, Romania, Northern Europe
Note: middle
Blends well with geranium, juniper, lavender, rose and sandalwood

Frankincense (*Boswellia thurifera*)

Principal properties: calming, cooling, decongestant, emotional, expectorant, rejuvenating, skin care, tonic
Treatment route: bath, compress, inhalation and massage
Specific contraindications: none known
Countries of origin: China, Ethiopia, Somalia, Arabia
Note: base
Blends well with: black pepper, lavender and sandalwood

Ginger (*Zingiber officinalis*)

Principal properties: analgesic, antibacterial, antiemetic, anti-inflammatory, antioxidant, antimicrobial, aperitif, aphrodisiac, carminative, cephalic, digestive, expectorant, rubefacient, stimulant, tonic, warming
Specific contraindications: none known, use well diluted to prevent skin irritation
Countries of origin: China, India, Japan, West Africa
Note: top
Blends well with: cedarwood, coriander, frankincense, neroli, patchouli, rose, rosewood, sandalwood and vetiver

Lavender (*Lavandula angustifolia*)

Please note that there are about 30 different lavenders currently on the market so that it is difficult to identify just what is being bought. Buy only where the botanical name is given. (This oil is said to be the most precious of all the essential oils because it is deemed to be useful for most conditions.)

Principal properties: analgesic, antibacterial, antifungal, anti-inflammatory, antidepressant, antiseptic, antispasmodic, balancing, calming, cardiotonic, emmenagogue, healing, hypotensor, rejuvenating, skin care
Treatment route; bath, compress, inhalation and massage (with caution neat for first aid purposes – stings and bites – 1 drop only)
Specific contraindications: none known
Countries of origin: France, Italy, UK, Tasmania
Note: middle
Blends well with: black pepper, citrus oils, clary sage, geranium, marjoram, neroli, and rosemary

Lemon (*Citrus limonum*)

Principal properties: antibacterial, anti-inflammatory, antirheumatic, antiseptic, carminative, digestive, disinfectant, diuretic, expectorant, sedative, styptic, vermifuge
Treatment route: bath, compress, inhalation and massage
Specific contraindications: none known, caution required with sensitive skin as may cause sensitivity, known phototoxic
Countries of origin: Australia, North and South America
Note: top
Blends well with: other citrus oils, cedarwood, geranium, eucalyptus, fennel, juniper, lavender, neroli, sandalwood and ylang ylang

Marjoram – sweet (*Origanum marjorana*)

Principal properties: analgesic, antibacterial, antifungal, carminative, cell proliferant, disinfectant, diaphoretic, diuretic, digestive, expectorant, hypotensor, laxative, respiratory, sedative, stomachic, tonic
Treatment route: bath, compress, inhalation and massage
Specific contraindications: none known
Countries of origin: France
Note: middle
Blends well with: bergamot, cedarwood, chamomile, cypress, eucalyptus, grapefruit, lavender, peppermint, rosemary and tea tree

Myrrh (*Commiphora myrrha*)

Principal properties: anti-inflammatory, antiseptic, healing, rejuvenating, respiratory, skin care
Treatment route: bath, compress, inhalation and massage
Specific contraindications: during pregnancy (a member of staff perhaps!)
Countries of origin: Somalia, North Africa, Ethiopia
Note: base
Blends well with: bergamot and lavender

Neroli bigarade (*Citrus aurantium*)

Principal properties: aphrodisiac, antibacterial, antidepressant, anti-infectious, anxiolytic, circulatory, digestive, neurological, skin care and sedative
Treatment route: bath, compress, inhalation and massage
Specific contraindications: none known but care needed with sensitive skin
Countries of origin: France, Egypt, Italy Morocco
Note: base
Blends well with: other citrus oils, jasmine and rose

Peppermint (*Mentha piperita*)

Principal properties: analgesic, antibacterial, antifungal, anti-infectious, anti-inflammatory, antispasmodic, carminative, cooling, decongestant, digestive stimulant, expectorant, hypertensor, insect repellent, mucolytic, neurotonic, tonic
Treatment route: bath, compress, inhalation and massage
Specific contraindications: none known, may irritate sensitive skin, in high dilutions may cause sleep disturbance or headache, acts as an antidote to homeopathic medicine, therefore store separately
Countries of origin: China, Europe, America
Note: middle
Blends well with: cajuput, lavender and rosemary

Roman chamomile (*Anthemis nobilis*)

Principal properties: analgesic, antibacterial, antidepressant, antifungal, anti-inflammatory, antiseptic, astringent, carminative, digestive, febrifugal, sedative, tonic, vulnerary

Treatment route: bath, compress, inhalation and massage
Specific contraindications: may cause dermatitis in some people (skin test prior to use recommended)
Countries of origin: England, France, Bulgaria, Hungary
Note: middle
Blends well with: bergamot, clary sage, jasmine, lavender, neroli, patchouli and rose

Rose (*Rosa damascena*)

Rose is very expensive because it takes 2000 petals to produce 1 drop of rose oil!

Principal properties: analgesic, antibacterial, antidepressant, antifungal, anti-inflammatory, antiseptic, antiviral, aphrodisiac, cosmetic, deodorant, disinfectant, diuretic, emmenagogue, germicidal, hepatic, sedative tonic, vulnerary
Treatment route: bath, compress, inhalation and massage
Specific contraindications: may cause dermatitis in rare cases (skin test recommended prior to treatment)
Countries of origin: Bulgaria, Turkey, Tunisia, China, India
Note: base
Blends well with: bergamot, black pepper, chamomile, fennel ginger, jasmine, neroli, patchouli, sandalwood, vetiver and ylang ylang

Rosemary (*Rosemarinus officinalis*)

Principal properties: analgesic, antibacterial, anticatarrhal, antifungal, antiseptic, expectorant, digestive, antidepressant, hypertensor, mucolytic, skin care, tonic
Treatment route: bath, compress, inhalation and massage
Specific contraindications: some advise caution with epilepsy, hypertension and asthma, may also irritate sensitive skin (advise skin test prior to use)
Countries of origin: Spain
Note: top to middle
Blends well with: cedarwood, lavender, marjoram, neroli, tangerine and thyme

Sandalwood (*Santalum album*)

Principal properties: antiseptic, aphrodisiac, antibacterial, antidepressant, antifungal, anti-inflammatory, antiseptic astringent, carminative, disinfectant, diuretic, emotional, expectorant, sedative, skin care, stimulant, tonic
Treatment route: bath, compress, inhalation and massage
Specific contraindications: none known
Countries of origin: India, Indonesia
Note: base
Blends well with: bergamot, black pepper, clove, jasmine, lavender, patchouli and rose

Tea tree (*Melaleuca alternifolia*)

It is considered a must in every first aid box, because of its low toxicity and immense versatility.

Principal properties: analgesic, antibacterial, antifungal, anti-infectious, anti-inflammatory, antiparasitic, antiseptic, antiviral, immunostimulant, neurotonic, skin care
Treatment route: bath, compress, inhalation, massage and mouthwash (gargle)
Specific contraindications: none known
Countries of origin: Australia
Note: top
Blends well with bergamot, lavender and myrrh

Ylang ylang (*Cananga odorata*)

Known as 'poor man's jasmine'.

Principal properties: antidepressant, antiseptic, aphrodisiac, balancing, calming, euphoric, hypotensor, reproductive tonic, sedative, skin care
Treatment route: bath, compress, inhalation and massage
Specific contraindications: none known
Countries of origin: south-east Asia
Note: top
Blends well with: citrus oils

Hazardous essential oils

There is some debate about which essential oils are safe to use. Although some of the following oils may be used in treatments by a qualified aromatherapist, it is generally felt that they should not be used by the layperson because of their potential to irritate the skin or cause toxicity:

Ajowan, almond (bitter), aniseed, balsam (Peru), boldo leaf, bergamot, buchu, cade, calamus, camphor, cassia, cinnamon bark and leaf, clove bud, leaf and stem, colophony, costus, *croton, elecampane, fennel (bitter), horseradish, jaborandi leaf, mugwort, mustard, opoponax, origanum, pennyroyal, pimento leaf, pine (dwarf), rue, **sassafras, *savin, savory (summer), southernwood, tansy, terebrinth, thuja, tolu, turpentine (unrectified), verbena, wintergreen, *wormseed and wormwood.

*It is illegal to sell these to the general public.
**Not to be used in foodstuffs in the UK.

The following essential oils are expressly contraindicated in patients with hypertension:

Cinnamon bark, clove, hyssop, juniper, rosemary, sage, savory, thyme.

The following essential oils are contraindicated when exposed to sunlight or before using a sunbed:

Angelica root, bergamot (expressed), cedarwood, cinnamon, ginger, grapefruit, lime (expressed), mandarin, orange (expressed), patchouli, verbena.

Further reading

Brown D (1993) Aromatherapy. Headway Lifeguides. London: Hodder & Stoughton.
Davis P (1999) Aromatherapy: an A–Z. Saffron Walden: CW Daniel Co. Ltd.
Tisserand R, Balacs T (1995) Essential Oil Safety: A guide for health care professionals, Edinburgh: Churchill Livingstone, pp 227–235.

Appendix III
Additional information

Glossary of terms

Acupressure: the application of pressure to acupoints, using thumb and fingertip pressure to stimulate the body's healing powers.

Alexander technique: type of posture training, designed to encourage people to adopt improved movement and posture, which leads to general neuromuscular improvement and coordination.

Analgesic: relieves pain.

Anosmia: loss of smell.

An mo: Chinese system of remedial massage that aims to tone internal organs by rubbing and pressing specific body areas, which are said to correspond to these organs. Dates back to the Han dynasty and refers now to that practised by lay people for general relaxation purposes.

Anti-allergic: reduces allergic sensitivity.

Anticonvulsive: relieves fitting.

Antidepressant: counteracts sadness.

Anti-inflammatory: reduces inflammation.

Antirheumatic: helps rheumatic pain.

Antiseptic: inhibits bacterial growth.

Antispasmodic: relieves muscular spasm.

Antisudorific: counteracts perspiration.

Anti-toxic: counteracts poisoning.

Antiviral: inhibits viral development and activity.

Aphrodisiac: increases sexual desire.

Astringent: helps tissue contraction.

Atlantean: describes the sailors who were associated with the mythological legends of the idyllic lost island continent of Atlantis that sank in an earthquake. The Greek philosopher Plato first described it more than

2000 years ago. There is still debate about the exact geographical position of this island and also whether the legend was merely a moral fable.

Augmentation cystoplasty: this major surgical procedure involves the removal of a percentage of affected bladder that is replaced by bowel. After this some patients are able to void normally and others will need to undertake intermittent self-catheterisation.

Aura: this is the radiating energy field surrounding a living organism. Its colour, shape and strength are dependent on the individual, but sickness and activity levels affect it. It is also said to interact with neighbouring auras.

Ayurveda: a sacred, ancient Indian medical system, which is still influential in India today. Good health is dependent on the three forces of vata (air), pitta (fire) and kapha (water) being in harmony. The word comes from the Hindi *ayur* for life and *veda* for knowledge or science.

Behaviour therapy: a type of psychotherapy, based on the principle that behaviour is learned (modified) as a response to a stimulus. Developed by Joseph Wolpe in the early 1900s.

Biofeedback: an individual's ability to learn to control their own autonomic responses by the use of appropriate monitoring devices.

Carminative: reduces flatulence.

Cephalic: stimulates the brain.

Channelling: in this process the healer acts as a route through which an external source, such as healing energy, can flow.

Chiropractic: from the Greek *cheir* for hand and *praktikos* for done by. Developed by Daniel D Palmer in 1895 and based on the concept that small subluxations (misalignments) of the spine can cause neurological defects and also internal organ disease. Treatment is by manipulation to restore the normal alignment of the spine and pelvis.

Cicatrisant: aids healing and growth of healthy skin.

Cholagogue: Stimulates bile production.

Cordial: acts as a tonic for the heart.

Counselling: this term covers a variety of techniques. Advice given may be specific or include psychotherapeutic approaches.

Crystals: stones (precious and semi-precious) said to emit energy and repel negativity. Claims are made that when used in therapy they generate healing vibrations, release blockages and correct energy imbalances. Sometimes the healer acts as the channel through which these energies pass.

Cytophylactic: encourages the growth of skin cells.

Deodorant: reduces body odour.

Depurative: cleanses the blood.

Digestive: helps food digestion.

Diuretic: increases urinary secretion.

Dowsing: in this instance means using a pendulum, etc. to locate and diagnose diseased organs or select a remedy (see Chapter 6).

Emmenagogue: balances menstruation.

Expectorant: anti-mucolytic.

Febrifuge: reduces temperature/fever.

Focusing: a technique that is adopted to enable individuals to become more aware of their inner self. This skill helps them explore their emotions and feelings and find the solution to their own problems from within themselves.

Fungicidal: inhibits fungal growth.

Gerson therapy: a dietary treatment, named after its developer, involving detoxification, the consumption of vast quantities of raw juices and nutritional supplementation; it is offered as an alternative approach to cancer care.

Haemostatic: stops bleeding.

Healing: a term that encompasses faith, spiritual and other healing styles, and involves the beneficial transfer of energy from one person to another.

Hepatic: acts as a tonic for the liver.

Homoeopathy: a therapy that uses medicinal substances and aims to treat like with like, developed by Samuel Hahnemann in the early 1800s.

Hoxsey: a cancer treatment developed in the 1840s by John Hoxsey, based on herbal teas, ointments and powders, and more recently immunotherapy and live cell therapy.

Hypertensor: raises blood pressure.

Hydrodistension: involves distending the bladder wall; used as a diagnostic procedure and also for symptom relief, for interstitial cystitis patients, by producing a degree of sensory denervation. This often needs repeating because symptoms may return.

Hypotensor: lowers arterial blood pressure.

Iatrogenic: disease occurs as a direct result of medical treatment. The term was coined by Ivan Illich and comes from the Greek *iatros* meaning physician and genesis for origin.

IER: International Examinations Board.

IFR: International Federation of Reflexologists.

Imagery: a technique of conjuring up mental pictures and using them positively to help alleviate pain, alter the pattern of a disease or attain personal goals (see visualisation).

Iridology: also called ophthalmic somatology, this is the study of the iris – all the bodily organs are said to be reflected in it. Jensen constructed a map of the iris in 1950 and it purports to show the relationship to all the bodily organs. It is used primarily as a diagnostic aid.

ISPA: International Society of Professional Aromatherapists.

ITEC: International Therapy Examination Council.

Laetrile: the Mexican pathologist Contreras, as part of his metabolic therapy, has promoted laetrile as a cancer cure since 1970. It consists of amygdalin (bitter almond) and, because it can produce cyanide in the body, is thought to be dangerous.

Laxative: aids bowel evacuation.

Laying on of hands: this involves the flow of energy from one person to another, with the intention to heal. Hands may or may not actually touch the recipient's physical body. Self-healing may also be activated by this. It is used in faith, psychic and spiritual healing.

Meditation: comes from the Sanskrit *medha* for wisdom. It is essentially a technique that may cover anything from prayer to the performance of elaborate rituals, for calming the mind. Some use a sound or phrase (a mantra), which is repeated silently or out loud to help focus the mind.

Megavitamin therapy: where large doses of vitamins are given to combat physical or psychiatric diseases. There is some concern that excessive use will cause toxicity.

Meridians: the main channels or pathways through which the Qi flows and where acupuncture points are located. The smaller channels are often referred to as collaterals.

Mistletoe: a parasitic plant, regarded as sacred by the Druids. Currently it forms the basis of Iscador treatment because it has been shown to have a cytotoxic effect, which may be useful in cancer treatments.

Naturopathy: a therapy that follows the principle that the body, given the right conditions, is able to heal itself. Modern naturopathy may involve many techniques and these include dietary and fasting measures, relaxation and, more recently, dietary supplementation and manipulation.

Nei Ching: the abbreviated version of the Yellow Emperor's Classic of Internal Medicine (*Huang Ti Nei Ching*), an ancient textbook, which describes the main principles of TCM.

Nervine: specifically acts on the nervous system.

Notes: this term, within aromatherapy, relates to the volatility (rate of evaporation) of an essential oil. Top notes generally evaporate rapidly, are highly volatile, and said to be uplifting and stimulating. Base notes evaporate more slowly and are believed to be calming, whereas middle notes are somewhere in between and tend to have balancing properties.

Osteopathy: works to correct faults in the structure of the body by manipulating and realigning displaced joints.

Placebo effect: a sense of benefit felt by a patient which arises solely from the knowledge that treatment has been given. Orthodox practitioners often suggest that complementary therapies work because of this rather than because they are therapeutic.

Psychic surgery: a dramatic type of treatment associated with the Espiritista church in the Philippines. The healers ('surgeons') 'operate on the patients, and as they move their hands over the patient blood may appear; yet there is no visible scar or cut. The benefits of this treatment have been anecdotally acclaimed but the therapy has never been meticulously analysed.

Qi (or Ki): pronounced as 'chee'; there is no corresponding word for it in the West. Loosely translated, it means energy or life force and is the active principle behind yin and yang balance. Health is said to be partly dependent on the appropriate flow and strength of Qi.

Radionics: the practice of using an instrument to diagnose disease and then to treat the disease at a distance using the radiaesthesic principles. The treatment will involve broadcasting healing waves with this radionics instrument.

Rebirthing: akin to psychotherapy, but where the patient is encouraged to relive their birth in order that any distressing events that may have occurred at that time can be ameliorated.

Rubefacient: stimulates capillary dilatation.

Sedative: calms nervous system.

Shark's cartilage: when processed, this is used as a supplement for cancer patients. Viewed with some scepticism by most orthodox practitioners.

Splenetic: tones the spleen.

Stimulant: stimulates sluggish systems.

Stomachic: tones the stomach.

Sudorific: induces perspiration.

Synergist: something that works in conjunction with something else to increase its efficacy (as in the blending of more than one essential oil to make a synergistic blend).

TCM (traditional Chinese medicine): a holistic system of medicine, which originated in China over 4000 years ago. Its underlying philosophy is that health is the balance of yin and yang energies, and disease manifests if this balance is disturbed by either internal or external forces. This is dependent on the appropriate flow of Qi.

Tonic: tones and invigorates.

Tricyclic antidepressants: these are given in smaller doses for patients suffering from interstitial cystitis than for those affected by depression, because they are thought to reduce pain, bladder spasm and inflammation.

Tsubo: surface points along the meridians, which correspond to acupuncture points. These are massaged during Shiatsu to stimulate the flow of Qi.

Tui Na: a type of professional clinical massage therapy, it comes from the Chinese *Tui* for push and *Na* for grasp. Tui Na applies pressure to specific points along the meridians to encourage the distribution and even flow of Qi through the body.

Vermifuge: expels worms.

Visualisation: this involves deliberately creating mental images with the conscious mind in order to evoke physical and emotional healing.

Vulnerary: heals wounds.

Yoga: is a personal system of health care, which may involve chanting, breath control and movement. It is from the Sanskrit for unity.

Useful addresses

Aromatherapy Trades Council (ATC)
PO Box 387, Ipswich, Suffolk IP2 9AN
Tel/Fax: 01473 603630; website: www.a-t-c.org.uk

Arthritis Care
18 Stephenson Way, London, NW1 2HD (Reg. Charity No. 206563)
Tel: 0800 289 170

Arthritis Research Campaign (formerly the Arthritis and Rheumatism Council for Research, Reg. Charity No. 207711)
PO Box 177, Chesterfield, Derbyshire S41 7TQ

Association for Continence Advice (ACA)
Winchester House, Kennington Park, Cranmer Road, The Oval, London SW9 6EJ
Tel: 020 7820 8113, fax: 020 7820 0442

Bristol Cancer Help Centre
Cornwallis Grove, Bristol BS8 4PG
Tel: 0117 980 9500 (provides support for patients and education for practitioners)

British Holistic Medical Association
59 Lansdowne Place, Hove, East Sussex BN3 1FL

British Reflexology Association
Monks Orchard, Whitbourne, Worcester WR6 5RB
Tel: 01886 821207

Continence Foundation
307 Hatton Square, 16 Baldwins Gardens, London EC1 7RJ
Tel: 020 7404 6875

Foundation for Integrated Medicine
International House, 59 Compton Road, London N1 2YT
Tel: 020 76881881; email: enquiries@fimed.org

Interstitial Cystitis Association (ICA)
PO Box 1553, Madison Square Station, New York, USA
website www.ichelp.com

Interstitial Cystitis Support Group (ICSG)
76 High Street, Stony Stratford, Buckinghamshire MK11 1AH

Multiple Sclerosis (MS) Research Trust
Spirella Building, Bridge Road, Letchworth, Herts SG6 4ET
Email: info@msresearchtrust.org.uk

NHS Careers
For information on courses
England: 0845 6060655
Ireland: 028 9023 8152
Scotland: 0131 226 7371
Wales: 029 2026 1400

Professional organisations

Association of Massage Practitioners
101 Bounds Green Road, London N22 4DF

Association of Medical Aromatherapists
11 Park Circus, Glasgow, Scotland G3 6AX
Tel: 0141 332 4924

Aromatherapy Organisations Council (AOC)
PO Box 19834, London SE25 6WF
Tel: 020 8251 7912; fax: 020 8251 7942; website: www.aromatherapy-uk.org

Institute for Complementary Medicine
PO Box 194, London SE16 7QZ
Tel: 020 7237 5165; email: icm@icmedicine.co.uk

International Society for Professional Aromatherapists (ISPA)*
ISPA House, 82 Ashby Road, Hinckley, Leics LE10 1SN
Tel: 01455 637987; email: admin@the-ispa.org; website: www.the-ispa.org
Publishes the journal *Aromatherapy World* quarterly.

Register of Qualified Aromatherapists (RQA)*
PO Box 3431, Danbury, Chelmsford, Essex CM3 4UA
Tel: 01245 227957; fax: 01245 222152

Shiatsu Society
Barber House, Storeys Bar Road, Fengate, Peterborough PE1 5YS
Tel: 01733 758341

**United Kingdom Central Council for Nursing, Midwifery and
Health Visiting (UKCC)**
23 Portland Place, London W1N 4JT
Tel: 020 7637 7181; fax: 020 7436 2924; website: www.ukcc.org.uk
Due to be replaced by Nursing and Midwifery Council (NMC) in April
2002.

Specialist fora

Royal College of Nursing (RCN)
20 Cavendish Square, London W1M 0AB
Tel: 020 7647 3333; website: www.rcn.org.uk
The RCN has published *Turning Initiative into Independence*, which is a list of
university and English National Board (ENB)-validated complementary
therapy courses for nurses. This is available from RCN Direct on 0845
7772 6100.

RCN Complementary Therapies in Nursing Forum
Tel: 020 7647 3763
Newsletter: *In Touch*
RCN Forum for Nurses working with Older People
Tel: 020 7647 3751

---

*Currently negotiating to form one united organisation. The International Federation of
Aromatherapists (IFA) are also involved.

RCN Forum Mental Health and Older People's Nursing Forum
Tel: 020 7647 3751

United Kingdom Central Council for Nursing, Midwifery and Health Visiting (UKCC)

23 Portland Place, London W1N 4JT
Tel: 020 7333 6541/6550/6553; fax: 020 7333 6538
Professional advice service email: advice@ukcc.org.uk
Publications: fax: 020 7436 2924; email: publications@ukcc.org.uk

Suppliers of essential oils, etc.

Circaroma Ltd

45 Foulden Road, London N16 7UU
Tel: 020 7249 9392; fax 0870 134 7785; email: Circaroma@aol.com
Producers of handmade organic skincare – may be personalised for individual therapists.

Denise Brown, Beaumont College of Natural Medicine

MWB Business Exchange, 23 Hinton Road, Bournemouth, Dorset BH1 2EF
Tel: 01202 708887; website info@beaumontcollege.co.uk
Provides courses in massage, aromatherapy, reflexology, etc., and sells oils to qualified aromatherapists

Essentially Oils Ltd

8–10 Mount Farm, Junction Road, Churchill, Chipping Norton, Oxfordshire OX7 6NP
Tel: 01608 659544; email: sales@essentiallyoils.com – excellent monthly newsletter available by mail or on website: www.essentiallyoils.com

Government and independent publications

Complementary and Alternative Medicine (CAM) (2000) 6th report from the House of Lords Select Committee on Science and Technology (HL Paper 123). London: Stationery Office.

Text available from Parliamentary website: www.publications.uk/pa/id/idsctech.htm

Complementary Medicine (2000) Information pack for primary care groups.

Produced collaboratively by the Department of Health (DoH), Foundation of Integrated Medicine (FIM), NHS Alliance and National association of

Primary Care – designed to act as a reference on the complementary and alternative therapies provided by primary care groups (PCGs) and can be downloaded from their websites (see below).

Health Education Authority (1996) Getting Active, Feeling Fit. London: HEA.

Help the Aged, Information Department (WIS)
St James's Walk, Clerkenwell Green, London EC1R 0BE
Provide free confidential Senior Line (0800 65 00 65) and leaflets on financial matters, housing, home, safety, and health issues (registered charity no. 272786).

Integrated Healthcare (1997) *A Way Forward for the Next Five Years?* London: FIM.

Discussion document published by the Foundation for Integrated Medicine on behalf of the Steering Committee for the Prince of Wales Initiative on Integrated Medicine (for website see below).

National Service Framework (NSF) for Older People (2001)

The first blueprint for the care of older people in England, which outlines eight national standards to improve care.

Available from:

NSF for Older People Implementation Team, Department of Health, 133–155 Waterloo Road, London SE1 8UG
Tel: 020 7972 3000; website: www.gov.uk/nsf/olderpeople.htm
The Standard Nursing and Midwifery Advisory Committee's report on the role of nurses caring for older people is online: www.doh.gov.uk/snmac.htm

Research into Ageing (ESTAR2)
4th Floor, 207/221 Pentonville Road, London N1 9UZ
Provide free *Focus on Healthy Ageing* leaflets, including dementia, breathlessness and falls (Reg. Charity No. 277468).

Additional internet sites

birchhillhappenings.com/aroma1.htm
email: albuddy1@aol.com
Although Alan Keay does not supply essential oils outside of the USA, he

does provide very informative regular aromatherapy newsletters, about the use of oils, via the email)

www.doh.gov.uk
Department of Health official site (provides press releases, research reports and links to other sources, including the European Union).

www.HealingOnline.co.uk
A holistic website created by a 'netpreneur' after his mother was successfully treated by a complementary therapist.

www.healingtouch.com

www.healthworks.co.uk
Provides daily medical and health news from around the world.

www.netdoctor.co.uk
Provides advice on health related issues, including diagnosis and prevention.

www.nhsalliance.org
NHS Alliance (provides very useful links to other sites).

www.patient.co.uk
Provides details of complementary therapies and their usage.

www.primarycare.co.uk
National Association of Primary Care.

www.purplehealth.com
Keen to promote practitioner referral services.

www.quackwatch.com
Takes a critical look at complementary therapies.

www.reutershealth.com
News archive (provides news, drug database, Medline and health information for both professionals and consumers).

www.thinknatural.com
Retail site (also provides information on herbal supplements, minerals and vitamins).

www.wellbeing.com
Boots the Chemist/Granada Television (includes information on complementary therapies).

www.who.org
World Health Organization: provides detailed articles on health issues/diseases.

Index

269